BIOTECH & PHARMACEUTICAL HAND BOOK

BIOTECH
&
PHARMACEUTICAL
HAND BOOK

by
P.K. Chattopadhyay
Working Experience
B.Tech. (F.T.B.E.), P.G.D. (F.T.B.E.) (J.U.)
In Production Quality Control Lab., Project Work,
R & D work with Nityakali Rice Mill & Solvents
Extraction Plant, Bengal Distileries Ltd.,
The Indian Yeast Company Ltd.,
Kusum Products Ltd.,
Asian Bio Food (P) Ltd.,
S.I.R.I., Parle Biscuits Ltd.,
Apex Silicated & Chemical Inds., (P) Ltd.
Hayward Research Centre, (Shaw Wallace Group)

NIR

नेशनल इंस्टीट्यूट ऑफ इन्डस्ट्रियल रिसर्च
National Institute of Industrial Research
AN ISO 9001 : 2000 Company
106-E, Kamla Nagar, Delhi-110 007 (INDIA)

Published by :

National Institute of Industrial Research

AN ISO 9001 : 2000 Company

Distributed by :

npcs

NIIR PROJECT CONSULTANCY SERVICES

AN ISO 9001 : 2000 COMPANY

106-E, Kamla Nagar, Delhi - 110007 (INDIA)
Ph. : 91-11-23843955, 23845654, 23845886 (M) 9811043595
Fax : 91-11-23841561 Website : www.niir.org
E-Mail : npcs.india@gmail.com / info@niir.org

I.S.B.N. : 81-86623-01-9

Price Rs. 1895/-
US $ 200-

CONTENTS

1 ENZYMES

Introduction

The Student of Biology or Biochemistry will already have learned of the Universal association of enzymes with living matter and the important part played by them in all types of vital activity.

Enzymes are proteinous in nature.It acts with different substrate to produce small molecules to smallest molecule according to the reaction parameters like pH, temp, pressure and physical condition of the substrate.

All the enzymes are not capable to react alone with substrate to convert product. Sometimes there is requirement of presence of heavy metals like iron as iron ion, cobalt as cobalt ion or organic molecules which are called co-factors.

There are two types of enzymes according to their sphere of action:

(1) Exo-enzymes (2) Endo-enzymes.

Exo-enzymes are such enzymes which are produced outside of the cells and react with substrate to convert product.

Endo-enzymes are such enzymes which stimulate inside the cells and convert substrate to product, inside the cells.

Basically enzymes are like organic catalyst produced by living cells. Live catalyst enzymes are capable of accelerating chemical reaction by millions of times under normal room temperature in 'soft' solvents. They have another quite unique ability-strict selectiveness in the presence of definite enzyme only one, the only one, of all possible reactions will, as a rule proceed.

Manufacturing Process

Basically major enzymes are produced by microbial fermentation process. Microbes may be bacteria, yeast or mold, it may be some times plant origin.

Production of α - Amylase (By Bacterial use) :-

Medium Composition :

Soluble starch	55.25%
K_2HPO_4	2.76%
Yeast Extract	13.81%
Peptone	27.6%
$MgSO_4$ $7H_2O$ .25	0.55%

The above composition ingredients dissolve in 25 times of water and sterilised at 115°C for 15 minutes. A Solution of 10% Sodium Carbonate in water was also sterilised at 115°C for 15 minutes . These two solutions were mixed to prepare a culture medium 250 ml in 1 litre Shake flask. Use inocculum of Bacillus species NO- 38-2 (A.T.C.C.21783). Make medium pH-10 and shake culture at 37°C for 48 Hours. The cells were removed from the culture by a centrifuge and at pH-9, 1ml. of this culture filtrate contained 2500 units of Alkaline amylase.

This culture broth throughly cooled and 3 volumes of acetone were added by which enzyme precipitated quantitatively. This precipitate was throughly washed with acetone and dried in air. About 11 grams brown powder were obtained from the 1 litre of the culture broth. The samplc obtained thereby has an optimum pH around 9.0 and it was found to be an amylase. (Specific Activity 200,000 u/gm).

Manufacturing Process of Fungal α- amylase :

The mold is cultivated on a nutrient medium containing the following composition

Starch	-	50 - 90 gms/litre
$NaNO_3$	-	8 - 15 gms/litre
$MgSO_4$	-	0.4 - 1.5 gms/litre
KH_2PO_4	-	0.2 - 1.2 gms/litre
KCL	-	0.5 gms/litre
$FeSO_4$	-	0.001 - 0.08 gms/litre
$Mg(NO_3)_2$	-	0.2 - 0.8gms/litre
$Mg(H_2PO_4)_2$	-	0.1 - 0.7.gms/litre

20% extract of Malt sprouts 20% by volume.

Preparation of seed culture :

Commercial viable strain of Aspergillus oryzae is grown in a test tube containing nutrient media 7ml (previously strilise). Growth of strain in test tube is washed by strile water and transfer to a shake flask containing a litre media of composition.

Starch – 60 gm, $NaNO_3$ – 9gm, $MgSO_4$ – 1.0gm, KH_2PO_4 – 1gm, KCl – 0.5 gm, $FeSO_4$ – 0.03gm, $Mg(NO_3)$ – 0.2gm, Mg (H_2PO_4) – 0.1gm.and 10% extract of malt sprouts 10% by volume.

The seeding culture is grown for 30 Hours on a shaker receprocating at a speed of 180 R.P.M. at a temp. of 30°C.

Commercial Process:

Now Produce seed culture (0.5%) is transfered in sterile conditon into a fermentation tank containing sterile media of composition.

Starch	-	80 gm/litre
$NaNO_3$	-	12 gm/litre
KH_2PO_4	-	1 gm/litre
$MgSO_4$	-	1 gm/litre
KCl	-	0.5 gm/litre
$FeSO_4$	-	0.3 gm/litre
$Mg(NO_3)_2$	-	0.8 gm/litre

$Mg(H_2PO_4)$	-	0.5 gm/litre

and 20% extract of Malt sprouts 20% by volume.

Fermentation time	-	72 Hours
Temp	-	30°C
Aeration Rate	-	9 c.f.m. First 24 Hr.
		18c fm-25-72 Hrs.

There will be foam in the fermentor which canbe controlled by antifoam odl like sperm oil or any other suitable antifoam oil.

After completion of fermentation my celium in the fermented broth be seperated by filtration or centrifugal separation.

The activity of α-amylase in the culture filtrate 20 units/ml. The filtrate is dialyzed with 0.03M Phosphate bufter at pH 7.15 for 12 Hours. The obtained dialyzed is divided into several equal portions containing 1000 mg of protein each and each having the activity of α-amylase of 10,000 units. Each portion of the dialyzed is passed through an individual column packed with 10 gm of diethyl amine ethyl cellulose. The diameter of the column is 35 m.m., the height 250 m.m. During this operation α-amylase and other proteins are absorbed on the column packing.

Next the α-amylase is eluted from the sorbert. The process is carried out in two steps. The first elution is effect with 0.06 M phosphate buffer at pH-7.15. During this operation only the accompanying proteins are eluted where as the α-amylase remains on the column packing.

α-amylase is eluted during the 2nd step when 0.11M phosphate buffer at pH-7.15 containg 0.001M solution of calcium chloride is passed through the column. The buffer completely elutes the fraction containig α-amylase.The field of α-amylase is 300mg having total activity of 10,000units that is the yield of α-amylase after elution is 100%.

Dialysis, adsorption and elution of protein is carried out at a temperature of +8°C. The specific activity of α-amylase obtained according to this process was almost twice as great compared with the activity of α-amylase obtained by the known method.

The activity of the product is expressed in international units (I.U.). This is expressed in I.U/cc^3 when the product is in solution and in I.U/gm when the product is solid.

Stabilisation of α - amylase :

Bacterial α-amylase can be stabilise in presence of Sodium and Calcium salts in solution(especially Calcium Acetate).

β - Amylase :

β-amylase the saccharifying enzymes produces maltose from starch, glycogen dextrins by selectivity removing maltose units at the nonreducing ends of the molecule chains, β-amylase activity also stops at the α-D(1→6) branching linkages of amylopectins leaving polysaccharides termed limited dextrins.

Manufacturing process by using Bacterial Culture :

A medium containing 5% milk casein, 2% corn steep liquor, 10% soluble starch and enough water to make 15litres was sterilized in Jarfermentor, adjusted to pH 7.0-7.2 and inoculated with commercial viable strain of B Megaterium. The mixture was incubated at 30°C for 2days with stirring where upon the broth showed an enzyme activity of 25.5 unit/ml.

The culture was centrifuged at 8000 r.p.m. for 20 minutes to remove the cells and the supernatant was mixed with enough solid $(NH_4)_2SO_4$ to precipitate a crude enzyme product. It was dissoled in M/100 acetate buffer solution and the solution was dialyzed against running tap water for 3days. Impurities still present were precipitated by adding 25% lead acetate solution drop by drop. The precipitate was removed by centrifuging.

The enzyme was again salted out with $(NH_4)_2SO_4$, dissolved in M/100 acetate buffer at pH-6 and the solution was heated 15' at 60°C. It was dialyzed and enzyme from the further purified solution was absrobed on a molecular sieve chromatographic medium (SE Sephadex G-25), eluted with M/2 sodium chloride solution and get filtered to Sephadex G-100. The active fraction was freeze dried and thus product dried β- amylase obtained activity of 100 units per mg and thus had 50% of the original broth.

Pectolytic Enzyme :

This enzyme is prepared by solid state fermentation using mold strain of commercial viable.

Preparation of culture :

Took commercial viable strain of Aspergillus Carbarierius transfer to sterile test tube containing nutrient Agar medium, then plate (Petridish) it to grow pure individual colony and then pick up well defined colony and transfer it to a test tube containing liquid nutrient media. Keep it for 24hrs at 37°C and then transfer it to shake flask containing 250ml solid nutrient media and keep it for growth of 24hrs. This growth is used as seed culture for the propogation.

Manufacturing Process :

Took wheat bran,add to it 0.5-2.0% organic nitrogen source, and acidic mineral salt solution. Sterilise the media and put the media mixture in perforated plastic trays (Tray's dimension = 60cm × 40cm × 10cm) of depth 5cm and then sprayed the inocculum spores 0.5% – 1.0% on the trays. Put the trays in fermentation room with allowing steril air flow rate 12 c.m.f., with RH% in the room 70 – 90 and temperature of room 28°C-32°C and time of fermentation will be 24-30hrs.

When the fermentation will be completed fermented materials are taken out and extract out the enzyme by water extraction process.Fermented material took in a extractor and extractor base will be perforated according to flow rate of liquid, liquid collected in a vessel from wnich extracted liquid will be circulated by pump. Extracted liquid contents enzyme which will be clarified by centrifugation (bowl type centrifuge) process.Clarified liquid is then collected in a vessel and enzyme precipitated by addition of ethyl alcohol at low temperature of 8°C.Then seperate out enzyme by filteration process. Dried it by freeze drying process. Keep the poweder in cool place prefrably at 4°C temp.

Invertase

It is prepared from yeast. Yeast starain of saccharomyces uvarum or saccharomyces cerevisiae grown in mannnose media instead of sucrose media will be enriched by invertate or grown in excess of sucrose media.

Invertase concentrate is prepared from yeast by plasmolysis the cells and allowing auto lysis to occur. Plas molyzing agents are ether, $CHCl_3$, toluene ethylacetate, benzeen, xylene, carbondisulphide, corbon tetra chloride, amyl alcohol. Which reduce the surface tension of water. plasmolysis done at pH 10-12 at 30°c.

Enzyme which is produce purified by adsorption Technique or by precipitation Technique. For adsorption technique bentonite, Znic sulfide, calcium Phosphate or aluminium hydroxide can be used and also many other substance can be used.

For precipitation strontium hydoxide, ethyl Alcohol, Acetone, $(NH_4)_2SO_4$ is used as precipitating agent.

Enzyme is seperated in the form of an adsorption complex with calcium phosphate and then precipitate is washed and dried at low Temperature. Invertase solution concentrated to a syrupy consistency is dried on glucose or lactose at low temperature produce white stable powder posses high enzyme activity.

Celluloses and Hemicelluloses :

Several types of calluloses are involved in the complete hydrolysis of cellulose. Consequently a commercial cellulose preparation should include all these components.

Trichoderma viride produced active cellulose and xylanase in solid culture using wheatbran, rice straw or news papers. These enzyme were also produced insubmerged culture using Aricel and wheat germ. pH of the media showed be 3 and temp. maintained 30^0c.

Lytic enzyme

Pelleculoria Sasakii or pelleculoria filamentosa may be cultivated either in a liquid culture medium or in a solid culture medium using known fermentation technique. Temp varied 15 – 4°c, and time of fermentation 48 – 240 Hours.

Manufacturing Process :

Commercial viable strain of pelleculoria sasakii is cultivated in sterilised media in shake flask. [media composition wheat bran 50%; Dried yeast - 2% water -48% media should be sterilised at 120°c for 20 minutes, culture grown at 28°c for 30-40 hours.

The resulting growth of the spore wath diluted by sterile water and used as commercial seed.

The solid media of above composition was starilised and put in plastic trays of depth 6cm, Then inocculate the previously growth inocculum to sterile media with aseptic condition. After complete inocculation media kept in fermentation room at 28°c-32°cfor 120 Hrs. at pH-4. Enzyme will be produced in the media is then extracted by an acetate buffer solution of pH-4 at ambient temp to completion of extraction. Now extract liquid was clarified by filtration and centrifugation process. clarified liquid content complete enzyme, now added aceton on the clarfied liquid to precifitate out of complex enzymes, the precipitate was filtered out and dried at low temp. This complex enzymes produced in the powder form. This enzyme preparation was found to be active to lyse the cell wall of a variety of micro organism including bacteria, fungi, yeast, Besid omycetes.

Stabilizers for lytic enzymes corboxy methyl cellulose (cm cc) sadium salt of CM.C, glycerine and monoethanoiamine can be utilised as stabilizing agent

These complex enzymes have the followring common characteristics.

(1) Active to lyse the living cells and dead cells.

(2) Lysing activity being stable in pH 3-9, Though optimum pH 5-7.

(3) The cell wall lysing activity optimum at 30°-40°c. But the optimum temprature varying depending on the nature of micro organism of which cells are to be lysed.

(4) Lysing activity of the enzyme become inactive at higher temperature then 50^0c.

(5) Cell wall lysing activity being inhibited by the presence of Mn^{++}, Ni^{++} or Zn^{++} ions.

(6) Exhibiting the enzymatic activity of cellulose, corboxymethyl cellulose, glucanasa, protease, hemicellulose and amylose.

(7) Being essentially compound of the component enzyme each having the molecular weights of at lease 50,000.

Proteolytic Enzyme :

(Protease) :

Protecolytic enzyme produces from Bacillus in suitable nutrient media are widely used in detergent industry.

Manufacturing Process :

Commercial viable Bacillus Firmus was cultivated at 30^0c on a rotary shaking table (220 R.P.M) in a 500 ml. flask containing 100 ml. media of the composition below. After 6 days of incubation the proteolytic activity of the culture was determined using the anson hemoglobin method, whose pH of the substrate adjusted to the appropriate value with NaOH.

Composition of the Media	–	gm/litre
Potato starch	–	40
Ground barley	–	100
Soyabean flour	–	30
Calcium Corbonate	–	5
Soyabean oil	–	0.5

The starch in the medium is liquified with α- amylase and the medium is sterilised by heating at 120^0c for 45 minutes After sterilisation, pH of the medium is adjusted to 9.7 by addition of ion of a 1M solution of sodium sesquicarbonate. After cultivation the enzyme activity of the broth determined at pH 7.5 was 50 Au /l (Anson unit per litre).

Recovery of enzyme

Liquid enzyme maybe prepared from the broth by evaporation at low temp or by reverse osmosis. Solid enzyme prepared by precipitation with salts such as sodium sulfate or with water miseible solvents, such as ethanol or acetone, removal the water in the broth by suitable drying methods such as spray drying may also be employed.

Micro-organism cultivation method

(Bacillus firmus.)

Dextrin	-	2.5%
Defatted soyameal	-	5.5%
Saccharose	-	3.0%
Na_2CO_3	-	0.9%
$NaHCO_3$	-	0.3%
Trisodium polyphosphate	-	0.3%
Temp	-	35-400c
Time in hours	-	50-60 Hours.
Aeration rate	-	Volume of air/volume liquid/ minute =1/2

These are different variety of protease yeild from different variety of bacterial strain (Bacillus species). Alkoline protease used in detergent industry.

Papain Concentrate :

Papyalatex is mixed with potasium metabisulphite in cold dimineralise water or distilled water, (water below 15^0c) stirred throughly and stored in a cool room for setling. The supernatantliquid is syphoned off and filtered. The clear filtrate is mixed with denatured spirit and allowed to settle in a cool room. The supernatant solution is decanted from the slurry. The slurry is filtred and the filtred cake is washed with rectified spirit where the solvent is remove by vaccum drying process. The semi dry cake is broken into lumps and dried in vaccum shelf drier. The potasium meterial is mixed with potasium metabisulphite and ground to require particle size. The powder papain concentrate is diluted with loctose powder for getting the desired activity.

General Process flow- Sheet

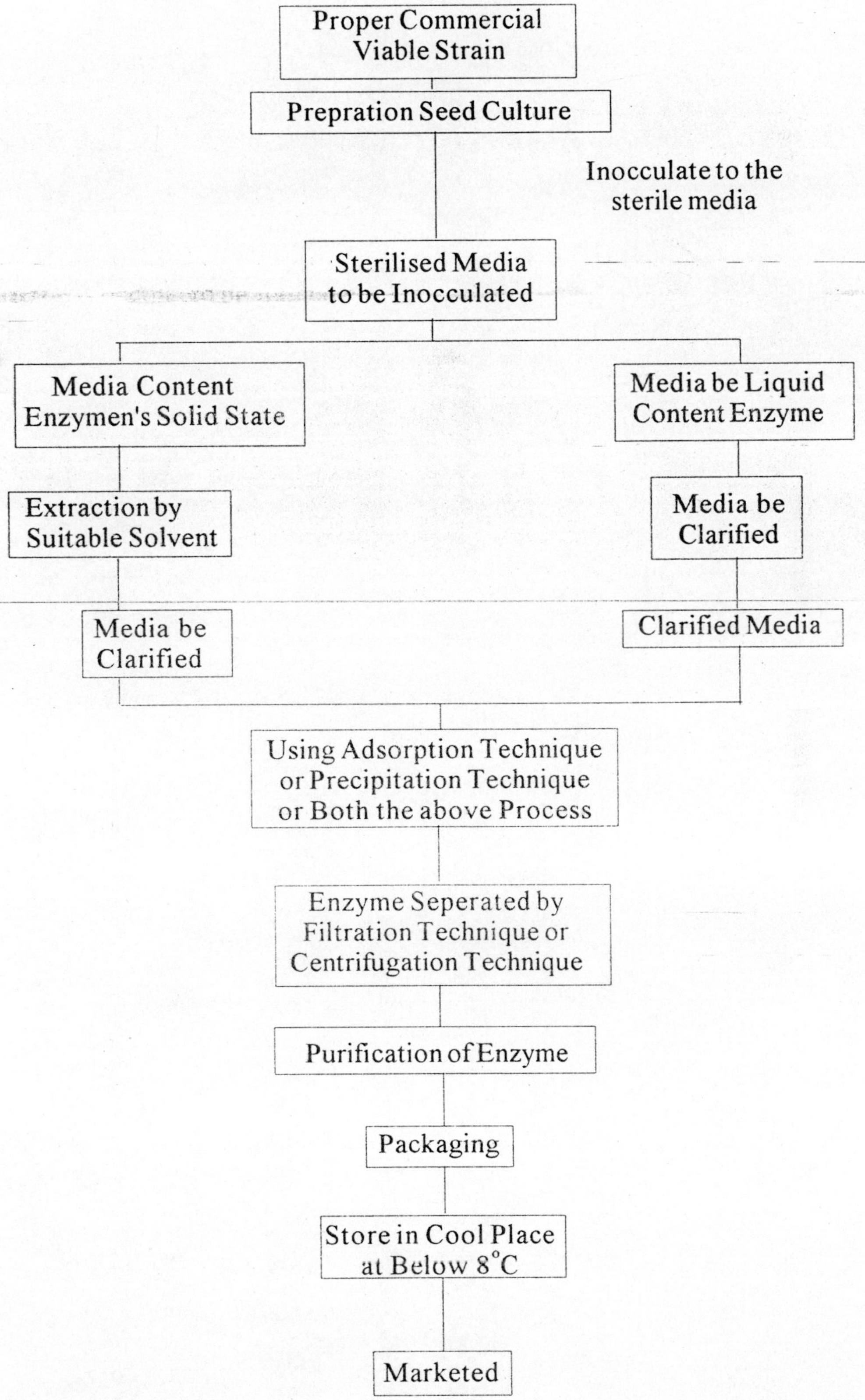

Generally Required Plant and Machinery.

1. Laminar Air Flow System.
2. Centrifuging machine.
3. Filtration unit
4. Drying unit.
5. Fermentation Room or fermentor.
6. Steriliser.
7. Refrigeration unit.
8. Extraction unit.
9. Settling unit.
10. Boiler.
11. Precipitation unit.

Test Parameters :

Assay of enzyme Activity.

Enzyme catalysed reaction can be monifored spectro photometrically, as many of the substrates or products of enzymes absorb visible or nonvisible light. This is the Commenst and simplest method of assaying enzymes. Spectrophotometry assay are especially common with enzymes that use nicotinamide co-enzyme that absorb at 340 nm in their reduced form.

Assay depend on (i) pH as a reaction Proceeds with pH meter, monitoring oxygen consumption or evolution during the course of a reaction using oxygen electrode or more generally following gas evalution with a monometer.

A standard and unit for enzyme activity is katal, defined as the amount of enzyme activity required to convert one mote substrate to produce per second.

In some cases it is more useful to express enzyme activity as the rate of change in solubility or viscosity of a material per unit wt or volume of enzyme added rather than inmore conventional terms such as the moles of products formed per mili gram of enzyme per second.

Enzyme Assay :

Iodometric Assay of Diastase (α - amylase) :

To determine the potency of the given enzyme taken diastase by the iodometry method.

Requirements :

Take enzyme diastase, o.1m Phosphate buffer pH = 7.0, 2% starch solution, iodine solution, 2% dextrin solution, 10 test tubes, 1 ml and 10 ml sterile pipettes.

Procedure :

1 gm of distase is to be weight out and make it serial dilution to 1:200, 1:500, 1:600, 1:700, 1:800, 1:900, 1:1000, 1:1100, and 1:1500, by phosphate Buffer solution of pH- 7:0.

5 ml of diluted iodine solution is pipetted into each of ten Test Tubes and are known as reagent blanks, 1ml of 2% dextrin solution is added to one of these and is taken as the reference standard : On mixing it gives a purple colour.

To prepare the substrate, 5 ml of diluted enzyme is added to 10 ml of starch solution. It is mixed and the time is noted. 1 ml of this is pipetted out at zero time and emptied in a reagent blank tube. After appropriate time intervals of 5, 10, 15 and 20 minutes, 1ml at the reaction mix is pipetted out into the reagent blank tubes till the colour of the Solutions matches the dextrin standard.

Composition of Iodine Solution :

Iodine 5.5gms and potasium iodine 11gm, This is dissolved in 250 ml of water 2ml of this solution is diluted to 1 litre with distilled water.

Compositon of Phosphate Buffer :

Prepare 0.02m Phosphate buffer by mixing sodium dihydrogen phosphate solution and disodium hydrogenpherphate solution.

The starch Solution should be prepared in phosphate buffer Solution.

Reading of the results -

The results are usually expressed as enzyme units. A unit may be difined as the number of milligrams of starch that can be Converted to the dextrin stage by 1ml of the enzyme in 1 hour at 30^0c and pH - 7.0.

The units can be calculated using the following formula.

$$\frac{a}{t} \times \frac{df}{b} \times 60$$

where a = amount of starch is mg in the reaction mixture.

t = Time Taken for the reaction.

df = Dilution factor

b = amount of enzyme the reaction mixture.

Polution Control :

Polution in the enzyme industry totally depend on the process parametes which is adopted by the industry. It may totally reduce the effuent out put from the industry.

Preservation of enzyme :

Enzyme can be store for long time at low temp i.e storing in plastic packaging at below 8^0c. in powder form. Use preservative with pure enzyme for enhancing the shelf life of enzyme.

In case of lytic enzyme C.M.C, Sodium salt of C.M.C, glycerine, and monoethanolamine can be used as preservative.

In case of amylase calcium Acetute or Sodium Acetute can be used as presevative.

Market

Enzyme are Biotechnology based produce of which (1) Alkaline protease (2) Nautral Protease (3) Other Proteases (4) Renins (5) Isomerase (6) Amylases (7) pectinases (8) Other carbohydrases (9) Lipase has very good demand in the Indian as well as in the international markets. Not any single enzymes can claims the very good demands but all of the above groups of enzyme has very good demand and future market increase 10 - 15% per annum.

Biotechnology

A perspective on world wide Market for Industrial Enzyme :

The curent world market for industrial enzyme is approximately $600 million (Sales Value). More than half of the market is in the U.S.A. The table (1) below gives details -

Table (1)

World Wide Enzyme Market

Enzyme		Market ($ million)
Alkaline Proteases	-	150
Netural Proteases	-	70
Renins	-	60
Other Proteases	-	50
Tsomears	-	45
Amylase	-	100
Pectinares	-	40
Other Carbohydrades	-	10
Lupares	-	20
Other	-	55
Total	-	600

Only small numbers of enzymes are used in large volumes. However today there are as many as 19 enzymes used in industry as described in brief in table (2).

Table (2)

Source and Applications of Industrial Enzymes

Enzymes	*Source*	*Application*
Bacterial α-amylase	B : Subtilis B : Li chenifomis	Starck lonversion
Fungla α-amylase	Aspergillus	oryzae Maltogenic Saccharificartion
Amyloglucozidase	Aspergillus	Strack syringes, Dextrose, Foods
Pullinlanses	Klebfiella Aerogenas	Debraneting Strack
B-Clulanose	B : Sublitis Penicillium amersonil	Brewing and Food Processing
Natural Protiens	B : Subtilis	Brewing/Flavouring
Neutral Protien	Aspegillus aryzae	Boiling
Alkaline Protien	B : Lichemiformis	Detergents
Cellulose	Trichoderma spp	Cellulose Hydrolysis
Invertose	Yeast spp	Confectionary
Pectinose	A : niger	Fruit/Wine Processing
Anthocyanose	A : niger	Decolouring Grapes
Rennet	Mucor spp	Milk Coogulant, Dairy Industry
Glucose Isomerases	Strep App	High Fructose, Corn Syrups

Lipase	Mucor spp	Dairy Industry, Detergent, Fat
	Aspergillus	Splitting
Lactose	S.Lactis	
	Kluyvsomyces	Lactis Dairy Industry
Hemicellulose	A : Niger	Baking, Fruits, Gums
Glucose Oxidase	A : Niger	Analytical Food Processing
Cataloase	A : Niger	Analytical Food Processing

Recent advances in γ-DNA technology engineering and process development have begun to influence the industrial enzymes market in a very positive way in recent yeast. These advances will continue to both lower the cost of enzymes and to improve the enzyme properties.

For instance the use of celluloses for processing biomors has until now been limited by high enzyme, sub-optimal ratios of activities and low specific activities. Improved charactrarization of this multi enzyme system of DNA mediated transformation system for filamentatous fungi and enzyme engg. have revitalized intrest.

Recent advance in enzyme engineering save introduced subtilism, chymosin, hyrolase, lipases, amylases etc. into commance. These are γ-DNA derived enzyme.

Uses

Amylases :

Use for the preparation of glucose from starch also it is used in the pharmaceutical Industry.

Alkaline Proteases :

Used in detergent industry for the Production of enzyme based detergent.

Celluloses :

Used for the hydrolysis of cellulose for further convnesion into sugar or alcohol.

Suppliers of Raw Materials :

1. PAA laboratries Inc
   13 Corporate plaza,
   130 Newport Beach,
   CA - 92660.
   Tel (714) 6408401.

2. BATTELLE
   505 King Avenue.
   Columbus,
   OHIO - 43201-2693.
   U.S.A.
   Tel. 614/424-5263.

3. Bio Business India Ltd.
   C-76, Fateh Nagar,
   Jail Road,
   New Delhi - 110018
   India.
   Tel. 091-11 - 5596820.
   Tex - 031 - 61922
   Fax - 091 - 115596820.

4. Sudhir Switch Gear Pvt. Ltd.
   305/6 Apeejay House,
   130 Bombay Samachar Marg.
   Bombay - 400023.

Suppliers of Plant and Machinery :

1. Sieco Engineers Pvt. Ltd.
   14/1 M.R.R.Road 2nd flour,
   Bangalore - 560002.
   Phone - 2238006.

2. Bio - Nics Equipment Pvt. Ltd.
   116 Dr. Radhakrishanan Road,
   Madras - 600004.
   Tel - 091-44-830512/13
   Tlx - 041 - 7489 S I P L N
   Fax - -044 -44- 830289.

5. M/S Vulcan Ltd., Mustafa,
   Dupodi Building,
   7A Sir P.M. Road.
   Bombay - 400038.

6. Dorr - Oliver,
   Hindustan Dorr - Oliver Ltd.
   Door Oliver House,
   Chankala.
   Andheri (East)
   Bombay - 400099

7. Chemical Engineering Corp.
   Chandra Building,
   Kalkaji Temple.
   Post Bag No. 8.
   New Delhi - 110019,
   Tel. 6439427, 6439318,
   Telephone - 84461

8. Buerau Wolf India Ltd.
   Pimpri, Pune - 411018,
   India.

9. Samarpan Fabricators Ltd.
   Plot No. A -182/A-183
   Lane Z, Road No 16,
   Wagle Industrial Estate,
   Thane - 400604,
   Tel. 505373/505630/505653.

Cost Analysis

(1)	Production : 1.5 Ton amylase per day.	
(2)	Fixed Capital Required :	
	(a) Land and Building	Rs.30,40,000/-
	(b) Plant and Machinery	Rs.75,00,000/-
	(c) Other fixed Cost	Rs.15,00,000/-
		Rs.120,40,000/-
(3)	Working Capital Required :	
	(a) Raw Matrial/3 Months	Rs. 60,00,000/-
	(b) Salary Wages/3 Months	Rs. 600,000/-
	(c) Other Miscllaneous Recurring Expense	Rs. 24, 00,000/-
	For 3 Months	Rs. 90, 00, 000/-
(4)	Total Capital Investment :	Rs.2,10,40,000/-
(5)	Project Cost :	Rs 1,42, 90, 000/-
(6)	Production Cost : (per annum)	Rs.4,07,30,000/-
(7)	Sales Turn over/annum :	Rs.4,95,00, 000/-
(8)	Profit/ annum :	Rs.87,70,000/-

(9)	Fixed Cost : (per annum)	Rs.19131000/-
(10)	BEP % :	68.56 %
(11)	% of Profit ratio on Total : capital Investment	41.6.8%
(12)	% Profit Ratio on Project Cost :	51.37%

2 ANTIBIOTICS

Theory

An Antibiotic is a chemical substance produced by a living organism that demonstrates inhibitory or germicidal activity toward micro organism in is inviro or invitro. It has been found also antimicrobial substance at produced by plants as well. The antibiotic Activity is sometimes referred to as being antibactirial, antifungal or antimicrobial.

Antibiotics are produced by certain fungi, bacteria, actinomycetes algea and lichens substances with similar properties are produced by some seed plants.

The most important and fertile source of commercially, important antibiotics is the genus Streptomyces of the actinomycetes. A large proportion of the antibiotics used in the fields of medicine and agriculture and food preservation.

The history of antibiotics abounds in critical situations. The euphoria which marked their appearence quickly gave place to a good deal of scepticism, follow by a notable expansion of the assortment of new drugs, while to-day, apparently , these are signs of a new upsurge, and all this within the space of half century or slightey more.

Invention of penicillin, saves the millions of life and wonder's of medical science, But now it is advice by the doctor's do not take any antibiotics without prior permission by the doctor since there is a certain adverse effect also produce by the antibiotics. The molecules of antibiotics in the form created by nature are by no means.

The discovery of antibiotics and their commercial production are considered as the most significant events of the current century in the field of medical therepy. Amongst the antibiotics penicillin was the first to be discovered and commercialised in early forties and even after over 40 years it continues to occupy a position of eminence having higher sales than any other antibiotic or group of antibiotics.

Semisynthetic antibiotics is much more active than normal synthetics antibiotics. New semisynthetic penecillin have been launched in mass production in the country. They may be subdivided into two basic groups, resistance to penicillinase and therefore, active against gram-positive forms of pathogens (mainly staphycococei) and antibiotics with a broad action spectrum the first group comprises methicillin, oxacillin, diachloxacillin, they have low toxicity and are well tolerated by most patient and are very effective in controlling a staphylococcal plage and other resistant pathogens cousing pneumonials lung abscesses, ostco myellite, sepsis. The therapeutic effects of methicillin and oxacillin are very close, but the advantage of the latter is that it may be administered not only by syringe but also by mouth, when the therapeutic concentration of the drug in the patients body is reduced.

The second group of semisynthetic antibiotic with a wide action range is represented, first of all by the popular ampicillin-active in regard of different groups of gram negative and grampositive micro-organism, Ampicillin has acquitted it self as a highly effective remedy for treating infections of the respiratary ways, kidneys and the gastro intestinal trach, the drug may be injected, and also be taken by mouth. It is well tolerated causing no side effects even in lasting administration. It is antimicrobial effect is enhanced when combined with antibiotics belonging to the group of so called aminoglu cosidase kanamycin gentamycin, and others. Thus the compoundampixo (a combination of ampicillin and exacillin) is

destru active to staphylococci, strepto cocci, the hemaphilic bacillus unfortunately ampicillin is unable to contact the blue pusbaciuus.

Semisynthetic antibiotics carbon penicillin to fight the pus bacillus, and also some bacteroids-strictly anaerobic i.e. living and developing in the absence of free oxygen and capable of causing accure inflammations carbenicillin has been successfully used for treating severe lesions in debilitated patients, including those with inflammation of the peretonium peritonites and grove leisons of the kidneys. Purposeful reconstruction of natural molecules will make it possible to produce ever more perfected kinds of semisynthetic drugs with enhance antimicobrial activity. Their importance in medicine without any exaggeration, is tremendous.

Some Antibiotics of proved value or of promise in the fields of medicine, food technology and agriculture.

1. Actinomycin	2. Amphoterecin	3. Anisomycin
4. Bacitracin	5. Condicidin	6. Carbomycin
7. Chloramphenicol	8. Chlortetracycline	9. Cycloheximide
10. Cycloserine	11. Erythromycin	12. Eulicin
13. Fumagillin	14. Griseofulvin	15. Neomycin
16. Nisin	17. Novobiocin	18. Nystatin
19. Oleandomycin	20. Oxytetracycline	21. Penicillins
22. Polymyxin	23. Puromycin	24. Ristocetin
25. Streptolydigin	26. Streptomycin	27. Subtilin
28. Tetracyclinc	29. Thiolutin	30. Thiostrepton
31. Vaneomycin	32. Viomycin.	

Some Problems of Research, Development and manufacture Relating to an antibiotic.

1. Isolation or collection of culture which is commercially stable and long self life.

2. Screening of cultures to detect those with antimicrotial activity.

3. Development of methods for submerged culture production

   (a) Development of Media

   (b) pH adjustment and control

   (c) optimum temprature.

   (d) optimum conditions of aeration

   (e) control of foam formation,

   (f) optimum time or lenght of fermentation.

4. Development of methods for isolation and purification

5. Determination of properties of antibiotics

   (A) Physical

      (a) solubility in solvents

      (b) Stability in acids, alkalie, heatetc

      (c) Adsorption and absorption

(B) Chemical

(a) Reaction

6. Evaluation of antibiotics

(a) Pharmacological tests.

(b) Toxicity in animals (mice, rats, guinea pigs, dogs, monkeys)

(b) Therapeutic effect on experimental infections.

7. Antimicrobial Action (spectra)

(a) Bacteriostatic Action.

(b) Bactericidal Action

(c) Fungestatic Action

(d) Fungicidal Action

General Manufacturing Process

The Process of antibiotic fermentation comprise mainly of the following steps.

1. Preparation of culture in laboratory.

2. Preparation of medium.

3. Preparation inoculunm in inoculator in the plant.

4. Antibiotic fermentration in the production fermentors.

5. Recovery of antibiotics.

6. Supply sterile air and sterile antifoam.

1. PREPARATION OF INOCULUM

Commercial viables strain selection is most important work from which first prepare proper culture which is further propagated to prepare seed culture.

Took a preserved commercial viable strain in test tube (which is called slant) or ampules. Strain transfer to test tube containing glucose media and keep it in the incubator at 30^0c for 24 Hrs.

Took test tube growth, and transfer small amount of growth in platinum wire loop and then streak it or previously sterile nutrient agar media or malted agar media in petridishes. Keep the streak petridishes in the incubator at 37^0 c and keep it for 2 days, colonies of the spores are developed, well seperated colonies are took out and put in a test tube containing glucose media or synthetic nutrient media keep the test tube for 24 hrs at 30^0c and then spread growth test tube over the sterile media in flask keep it for 30^0c for 24 Hrs, this growth be comes ready for culture for the preparation of seed.

Prepared culture is transfred to flask containing nutrient media and keep it on shaker at constant temp (30^0c) and the growth of the culture used as commercial seed for the commercial production.

Preparation of medium

For the preparation of medium stainless steel mixing tank of around 25M^3 is used. The tank is provided with agitators, steaming and aeration facilities. The raw materials used are starch, glucose, sucrose, and hydrol as carbohydrate source soyabeanflour, cotton seed flour, cornsteep liquor as natural nitrogen source, calcium Carbonate as a buffering agent, various sodium, ammonium, magnecium salts, oils and fats like groundnut oil, soyabean oil, lard falt, some micro elements are also essential ingredients of the fermentation medium.

The pre-weighed quantity of ingredients infixed proportion and standard quality are added to process water in the mixing tank. The volume is adjusted, pH is adjusted with alkali and heared to a definite temperature to sterile the medium (i.e 108°c for 60), the medium concentrate is pumped to main fermentation (All the attached line from media preparation to fermentor should be sterile) floor for further processing, though the basic raw materials are more less the same, but the exact quantities mixed are different for different antibiotics fermentation,where starch is used as carbohydrate source, it is first liquified with amylase before transfring to fermntor. The sequence of addition of raw matsials in the mixing tank is an important factor to arrive at the most nutritionally balanced medium

Propagation of inoculum in the plant

The inoculum potential ratio between inoculater and fermentor volume varies from product to product usually 5-10% inoculum is added, to the fermentor medium.

Inoculator is a stainless steel vessel with facilities of continous agitator, aeration and controlled temperature Being a small tank media, ingredients are added directly to it mixed properly, volume and pH adjusted and sterlized under steam pressure. After sterilisation, it is cooled to the desired temprature and kept under sterile pressure with steam sealing at every isolation value. Laboratory inoculine is brought from the laboratory and added to the inoculator aseptically. The cycle of in occulator is between 30-50 Hrs . The parametres maintain in the running inocculators are temperature to the optinum level which is different from different products continuous agitation and air flow usually one volume per volume of media. For maturitiy following is checked

(a) packed my celium volume

(b) pH

(c) Sterility.

(d) Growth characteristics.

If the above is optimum level, it is ready for transfer to the fermentor.

Fermentation in Fermentors

Media for fermentor is mixed in seperate media mixing tank. Prepared media concentrate is pumped to the fermentor. For sterilization of media different techniques are used :

(1) Batch sterilisation in the fermentor itself.

(2) External conditions sterilization with direct steam injection in a heating coloumn or with indirect steam in heat exchangers. The Types of sterilization and product, where external sterilization is done, cooled media is pumped to pre-sterilized fermentor which kept under sterile air pressure.

When the fermentor is ready with medium, inocculations transfred to it under sterile condition through sterile pipelines.

The period of fermentation in fermentor may vary from 5-15 days depending on the product taken. As most of the antibiotics fermentors are aerobic continuous agitation and aeration is carried out during fermentations sterile air is fed to the fermentors in controlled quantities for respiration and growth of the organism. Sterilisation of air is done by filtering it through pack glass wool filter or cotton filter or fine metalicmesh filters.

Inside the fermentor for oxygen transfer, the design of fermentor play very very important role.

During fermentation temperature is controlled by flowing chilled water through cooling coil or jackets, internal or external by outomatic control instruments.

Foam is controlled by addition of sterile vegetable oil / mineral oil/ silicon defoamers, in doses controlled by automatic foam control system.

During the cycle of fermentation control of pH is very important and is maintained at the optimum level by addition of alkoli solution or ammonia (gas or solution) by automatic pH control system.

A strict control on residual at nutrient level (carbon and nitrogen source) is maintained Throughout the cycle by giving continuous or intermitteat shots to the fermentor.

When the fermentation is over and maximum activiity has been achieved (it is a predetermined period), it is harvested and sent to filtration section.

Recovery of Antibiotics

Fermented broth after preliminary treatment is filtered organism in the form of mycelial mate is rejected and clear liquid (native solution) contaning antibiotics is further processed. For filtration conventional plate and frame filter presses are used or drum filters or notch filter are used.

The antibiotics from the native solution is recovered by precipitation or solvent extration or through in exchange methods depending on the antibiotic processed.

Manufacturing Process of penecellin

For manufacturing of penicillin especially used mold strain of penicillium notatum or penicillium chrysogenum which are commercial viable. A superior strain yielding about 99% penicillins.

Sporulation Media

In the production of penicillin, it is necessary to grow rapidly large numbers of spores for inocailation or seeding purposes.

Used sporulation mediums are :

(1)	Glyeerol	-	7.5 gm.
	Canemolasses	-	7.5 gm.
	(Ediblegrade)		
	Corn steepliquor	-	2.4 gm.
	$MgSO_4$, $7H_20$	-	0.05 gm.
	KH_2 PO_4	-	0.060 gm.
	Peptone	-	5.00 gm.
	Nacl	-	4.00 gm.
	Fe-tartarate	-	0.005 gm.
	$CuSO_4$, $5H_2O$	-	0.004 gm.
	Agar	-	2.5 gm.
	Distilled water	-	1 litre.

(2) For producing mold spores used fresh whole-wheat bread (free of mold inhibitor) is cut into I cm, cubes and steam strilized in shallow layers in Erlenmeyer flasks. The cooled bread is heavily inoculated with mold spores and incubuted at 25-27°c for 4-5 days After the bread cultures have partially dried, They may be stored at 40°c for as long as 2 weeks satisfactory. The spore covered bread may be crushed usually to a powderymass after 6-7 days and used for inoceulation purposes. As an alternative it may be mixed with 3-4 volums of a mixture of equal ports of sterilized whole whear flour and finely ground oat hulls.

(3) Wheat bran moistened with a 2% solution of corn steep liquor may also be used for sporolation media.

(4) Sporulation Media of the following composition also used :

Agar	-	15gm.
Sugar beet molesses	-	5.00gm.
Peptone	-	5.00gm.
Nacl	-	4.00gm.
KH_2PO_4	-	0.10gm.
$MgSO_4$, $7H_2o$	-	0.05gm.
Distilled water	-	1litre.

(5)	Sucrose	-	20gm.
	$NaNO_3$	-	6gm.
	KH_2PO_4	-	1.5gm.
	$MgSO_4.7H_2O$	-	0.5gm.
	Ca_2Cl_2	-	25gm.
	Water, tap or Distilled	-	1 litre.

Penicillin Can be produced by surface culture process or submerged culture process.

The spores of P. chrysogenum on agar slants are used to seed germination medium inflasks. After suitable period of incubation on the shaker, the contents are transferred from the shaker flask to special metal containers. The special container is aseptically attached to the seed tank and the mold suspenssion is forced into it through the use of sterile air under pressure. The mold from the seed tank is used as a starter for the fermentors. The cells concentration in the inocculum should be such that when it will be transfred to main frementor, cells concentration should be more than 1.5-2x106 cells/ml.

Raw Matrials used

Carbon source : Lactose, Cornstarch, Corn dextrin, glucose, sucrose.

3% - 6% solution of the above raw matrial may be used for carbon source for the production of penicillin, Nitrogen source. Sodium nitrate, ammonium sulfate, ammonium acetate and ammonium lactate, Corn steepliquor and other matrials.

Mineral source certain elements like phosphorus, Potassium, Magnesium, Sulfur, Znic and Copper beneficial for the production of penicillin. Some of the minerals are available in Corn steep liquor. Potasium and Phophorus are supplied as potasium dihyclogen phosphate, magnesium and sulfur as magnesium sulfate ($MgSo_4$ $7H_20$). Iron and copper when added in the medium, are usually suppiied as the sulfates. Zinc or manganes ions are presented optimum level in cornsteep liquor.

Corn steep liquor appears to contain adequate quantities of KH_2PO_4 and Mg SO_4-$7H_2o$. The use of Corn steep liquor in the fermentation medium greatly increase the yield of penicillin in surface culture and submerge culture fermentation. stimulatory effect of corn steep liquor is due to the presence arginine, histidine and glutamic Acid and possible to phenylacetic acid derivatives.

Precursors

Precursors are substance used in the production of antibiotics to increase the yield or to encourage the formation of a particular type of compound phenylacetic Acid used as precursor in penecillin frementation phenyl acitic Acid toxic at less pH, Toxicity can be over come by incrcating pH 5-5.8 before inocculation or by adding the phenyl acetic acid to the culture, after the pH has risen above tne critical value.

Amino acids such as α-cystine, α cysteine and valin appear to be important in synthesis of the beta-lactamethiozolidine ring system of the penicillins.

Conditioi. of the frementation

Temperature : Temperature of the media infermentor may varied from 24°C-30°C.

pH : Control of pH during the fermentation is essential, for too high or too low pH may result in considerable losses in penicillin. optimum pH. for penicillin fermentation may vary from 5-7.5.

The pH of the medium is influenced by the kind and amount of corbohydrate present, the amount of Corn steep liquor, the presence of buffers and other factors.

Carbohydrate are generally fremented with the production of some organic acids. Some carbohydrates, Such as glucose are fermented rapidly and tends to lower the pH level; other such as lactose are fermented more slowly and consequently the pH changes more slowly sugar feed rate of 0.03-0 .07 percent per hour is optimum.

Buffer agents : Maintain the pH within a range fovourable for penicillin production, calcium carbonate is widely used for the purpose.

Aeration : Aduquate acration required for the optimum production of penicillin. Aeration will be one volume\ of air or volume of media per minute.

Pressure : The use of pressure increate the effectiveness of earation. In the fermentation tank pressure may be varied 2ld / inch to 20 lb / in.

Increase the pressure to 40 lb/ in reduce the yield of penicillin.

Agitation : Agitation Requires varied from 50 R.P.M. - 500 R.P.M.

Antifoam agent

Antifoam agents are used for foam controlling in submerge fermentation used antifoam agents are tributyl citrate, 3%.0 ctadecanol disolved in lard oil, or soya bean oil. It is most important work to prevent contaimination of the medium used for penicillin production. Contamination usally produces rapid destruction of penicillin. In order to prevent contamination, it is necessary to sterlize all fermentantion tanks, pipe lines, and equipment with which the penicillin may come into contact. steam, for maline, caustic, savlon, etc used for strilizing agent of plants and area.

PRODUCTION MEDIUM

Synthetic media used for production of penicillin media compositions are as below wt/volume present.

Glucose	-	1%
NH_4So_4	-	0.04%
KH_2PO_4	-	0.75%
Na_2So_4	-	0.10%
$MgSO_4$, $7H_2o$	-	0.07%
$FeSO_4$, $7H_2o$	-	0.018%
$MnSO_4$, $_4H_2o$	-	0.005%
$ZnSo_4$, $7H_2o$	-	0.005%
$CuSO_4$	-	0.0008%.
$CaCl_2$	-	0.005%
$CaSO_4$	-	0.2%

The glucose was seperately sterilized in distilled water and added at the time of inocculation Additional glucose was fed to the medium during the Production phase at the rate of 0.03-0.07% and pH maintain 7.4.

Time of fermentation will be around 125-175Hrs. When the fermentation will be completed by checking of optimum yield of penicillin per ml of fermented broth. When the fermentation is completed, seperate mycellium by rotary drum filter or by contrifugation. Take fermented broth which contains penicillin. Now extract penicillin by using solvent acetone chloroform, ether, Amyloacetate and other solvent may be used, After complete extraction, extract liquid is pass through the ion exchange resin column so seperate out impurities or any foreign metal ions presant in it. After passing through ion exchange resin extract liquid is vaccum distilled at low temperature After words concentrate liquid goes through crystalisation process. After formation of crystal it is seperate out by centrifugation and wash completly, Then vaecum dried the crystals, After drying. Crystal pack is sterile container in aseptic condition.

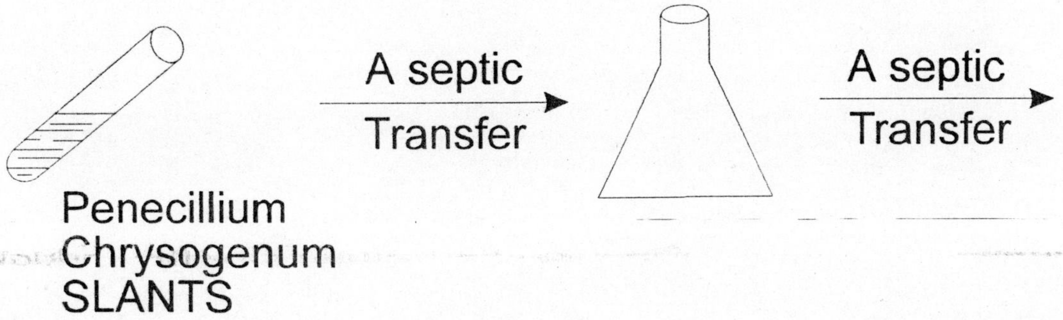
A septic
Transfer
A septic
Transfer
Penecillium
Chrysogenum
SLANTS

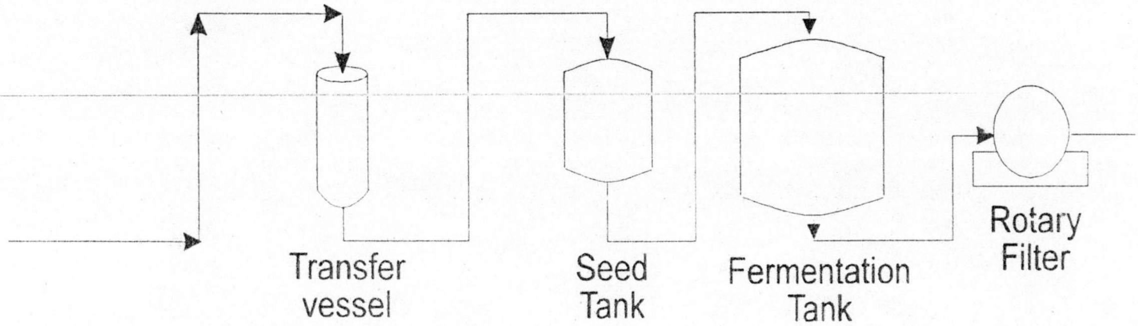
Transfer
vessel
Seed
Tank
Fermentation
Tank
Rotary
Filter

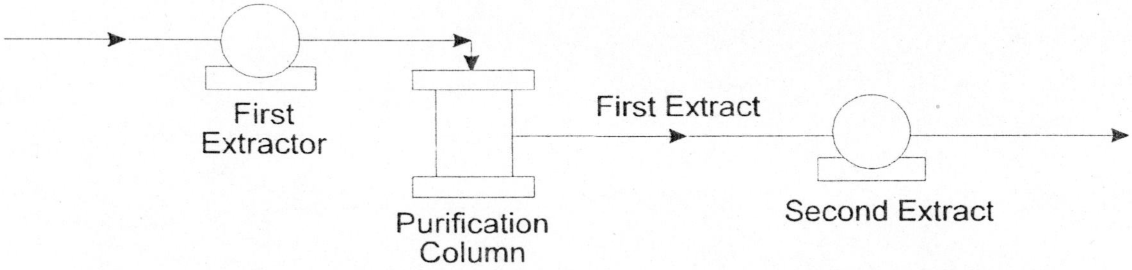
First
Extractor
Purification
Column
First Extract
Second Extract

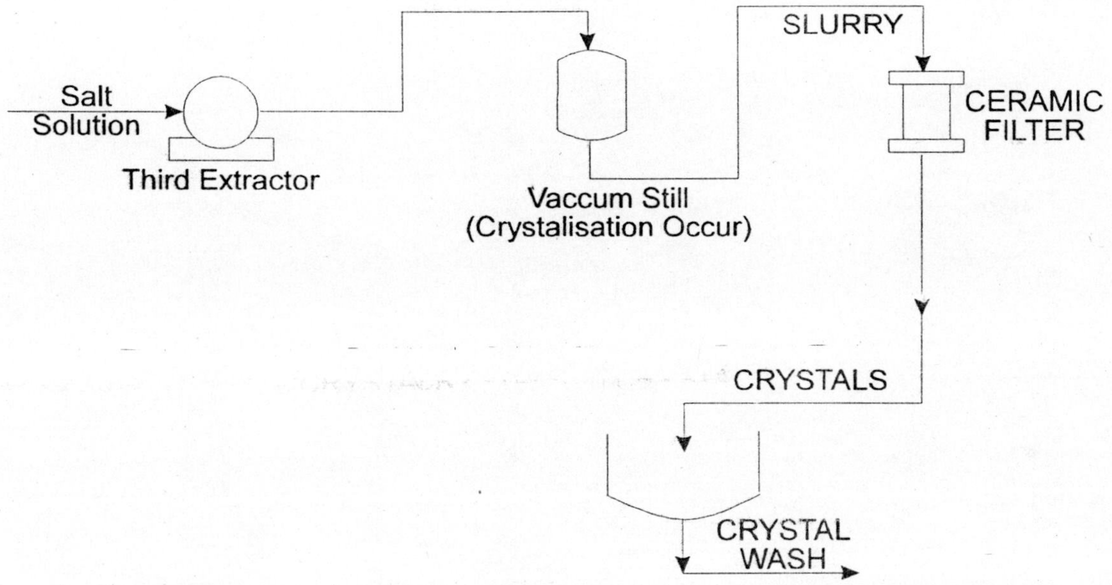
SLURRY
Salt
Solution
CERAMIC
FILTER
Third Extractor
Vaccum Still
(Crystalisation Occur)
CRYSTALS
CRYSTAL
WASH

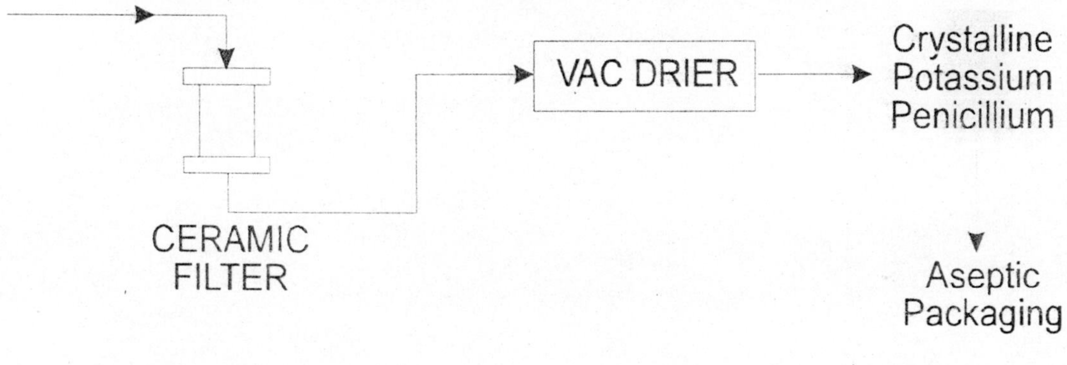
VAC DRIER
Crystalline
Potassium
Penicillium
CERAMIC
FILTER
Aseptic
Packaging

Properties of penicilline

Penicillin is active against certain gram positive bacteria in the presentce of blood, pus and body fluids.

It may be regarded as nontaxic, for very large doses may be administred over a relative long period of time without injurious effects. In a small percentage of cases individuals allergeic to penicillin are found.

Solubility

It is soluble in water. In acetone amylacetate, cyclohexane, dioxane, ethyl acetate, ethlyal cohor and ether, it is very soluble.

In benzene, chloroform and carbon tetrachloride it is less soluble.

Stability

It is very unstable compound It is stable only low temperature.

It decomposes by strongacids and alkalies.

It is inactivated by oxidizing agents.

Contact of heavy metals (Cuptor, silver, lead and mercury) destroy the penicillin, Znic salts also inactive penicillin. The antibiotic structure of penicillin destroy by penicillinase as enzyme secreted by a large number of bactria, molds and yeast.

It is necessary to use sterile media and aseptic methods during the production of penecillin and sterile water or other suitable diluents in the preparation of solutions of the solid matrial.

The crysalline salts of penicillin stable over a period of several months

Penicillin is much stable at the pH 6-6.5.

Reasonably stable pH range for penicillins 5.5 - 7.5.

The half lives of penicillins F.C, K and X are 11, 18.5, and 11 minutes, respectively at pH 2 and 24^{0}c.

Stabilizing Agent phosphate has a stabilizing influence on crude penicillin at 37^{0}c, The rate of lose of potency varied inversly the concentration of potassium dilydrogen phosphate present in the culture, medium at the begining.

Phosphate exerted stabilizing influence on sterile water solution of pencillin, which was independent of the buffering effect.

The Tetracyclines

The group of compounds includs chloro tetracycline, oxytetracycline, and tetracycline which are classified as broad spectrum antibiotic. In general the antibiotics of this group are active against gram positive and gram negative bectria and species of Ricetsia and prosses low taxicity.

Oxytetracycline

This antibiotic is also known as terramycin.

Manufacturing Process

Oxytetracycline is produced by S.R.mosus. It is amphoterie and forms a crystaline hydrochloride and sodium salt.

Carbon Source

Sugers, starch, or glycerol.

Organic nitrogen source

Soyabean meal, wheat gluten, cotton seed meal, lactalbumin, The enzymatic digest of casein or Tryptone, growth substances by distiller's solubles or yeast extract.

Minerals source

Sodium chloride, Potassium Phosphate, Magnesium sulfate, and Sodium nitrate.

Buffering agent

Calcium carbonate may be used as buffering agent.

Oxytetracycline (Terramycin) Produced by submerge fermentation process.

Fermenting media composition as below.

Soya bean meal	-	3%
Corn starch	-	0.5%
Enzymatic Digestcasein	-	0.1%
$NaNO_3$	-	0.3%
$CaCO_3$	-	0.5%
Vegetable oil	-	0.4%

The above ingredients are dissolve in tap water and pH adjusted to 7. The medium is sterilised for 1 Hour at 121°c and cooled to 28°c for seeding.

Aeration rate	-	0.5-2 Volume of air per volume medium per minute.
Agitation 100 R.P.M.	-	2000 R.P.M.
Fermentation period	-	8 – 10 days.
Temperative range	-	24 – 30°C.

At the end of fermentation titrevolume of media will be 1000 micro gram per ml.

Properties

(1) It posses low degree of foxixity.

(2) It is fairly stable is aguolever solution at about pH 2.4.

The structural formula of oxytetracycline as below.

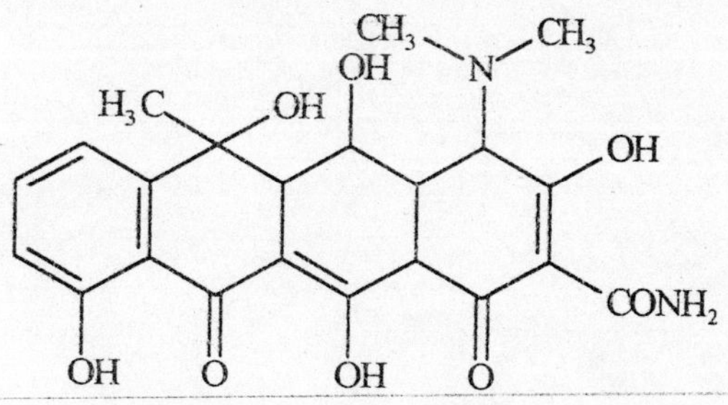

Test Parameters

Assays are carried out to determine the the potency of the antibiotic and test for sterility, toxicitiy, pyrogenicity, moisture and other items as may be required.

Potency of the antibiotic

A cylinder-plate method for determine the potency of penicillin as below.

Requirements of apprcatus

Ptridishes : 20 mm deep and 100 m.m. diameter.

Cylinder (*cups*) : The cylinders are made from stainless steel and have the followwing measurements. Outside diameter 8m.m. (+0.1mm) inside diameter 6mm (+.1mm) and length 10 m.m.(+ 1mm)

Standard stock solutions of penicilline (available in food and drug administration Department).

Phosphate buffer solution

Used for dilution of stock solution.

Preparation of plates

This consist of adding 21 ml. portion of uninoculated nutrent agar (Medium2) to sterile ptridishes allowring it to solidity, adding 4 ml. seeds agar to the surface of the base agar in each, plate, and dropping the cylinders on to the seeds agar.

The seeds agar is prepared as follows :

The test organism, which is carried on slants containing medium 1 and transfered once a week, is used to in occulate nutried broth (Medium 3). The broth culture is inchbated at 37°c. for 16-24 hrs. Two m uof this culture is mixed throughly with a 100 ml. portion of agar (Medium 1), which has been melted and cooled to 48°c four ml. of the seeded agar is placed on the surface of the base agar in each ptridish and spread uniformly by tilting the dish back and forth.

A suspension of the test organism which may be used over a period of a week, may be prepared instead of the broth culture for seeding the agar. The test orgamism is grown on an agar slant (Medium 1) at 37°c for 24 hours. The growth is washed by 2ml. of sterile physiological saline solution and transfered to a large surface of agar. The seeded agar is incubated at 37°c for 24 hrs and at room temp for 24 hrs. The growth on the surface of the agar is suspended in 50 ml. at sterile physiological saline, The suspension thus obtained is standardized" by determining the dilution which will permit 20% light transmission through a filter at 6500A° units in a photoelectric colorimeter" Fach 100ml portion of medium 1 is inoculated with 1.5-2ml. of the standardized suspension - Four ml. of the seedes agaris added to each ptridish containing 21 ml. of base agar, as described aove.

Four stainless steel cylinders are added to each plate, seperated by about 90^0 intervals on a radius of 2.8 cm.

Preparation of the sample

A stock solution of the sample that is being assayed may be prepared by dissowing it in sterile, distilled water.

Assay

A total of four ptridishes. each containing four cylinders. are used for each sample, two cylinders in each plate are reserved for dilution of the working standard and two for dilution of the sample. One cylinder in each plate is filled with a dilution of the working is filled with adilution of the working standard that contains 1 unit per ml of penicillin. A second cylineter in each plate is filled with a dilution of the working standard that contains 0.25 unit per ml. A third cylinder in each plate is filled with a dilution of the sample that contains an estimated 1 unit per ml. A fourth cylinder in each plate is filled with dilution of the sample that contains can estimated 0.25 unit per ml. The plates are placed very carefully in the incubator spaces and stored for 16-18 Hours at 37°c. After the incubation period, the diamenter of the zone of inhibition are measured so the nearest 0.5 m.m by means of a suitable measuring device, such as a clony counter contatining a measuring scale (in millimeters) etched into the glass that supports the dish over the light source.

Estimation of potency and Error

From the assay data the values of V and W are determined for each plate

V = (UL+UH)-(SL+SH) - (1)

W = (UH+SH)-(UL+SL) - (2)

SH = Diameter (in mm) of zone of inhibition of 1.0 unit/ml. dilution of the standard.

SL = Diameters (in mm) of zone of inhibition of 0.25 unit/ml of standard.

UH = Diameter (inmm) of zone of inhibition of test sample dilution 1 unit/ml.

UL = Diameter (in mm) Of zone finhibition of test sample at 0.25 unit/ml.

After the W and V values have been calculated, the point in the chart "A" that corresponds to these value is located and the potency aser tained from the radial lines.

The chart should not be used for determining the potency of a sample where is the potency is less than 50% or higher than 150% of the standard.

Medium 1

Peptone	-	6 gm.
Pancreatic digest of casein	-	4gm.
Yeast extract	-	3gm.
Beef extract	-	1.5 gm.
Glucose	-	1 gm.
Agar	-	15 gm.
Distilled water to make up volume	-	1 litre.
pH	-	6.5-6.6
		(After Sterilisation)

Medium 2

Peptone	-	6 gm.
Yeast extract	-	3 gm.
Beef extract	-	1.5 gm.
Agar	-	15 gm.
Distilled water	-	1 litre.
pH	-	6.5-6.6
		(After sterilisation)

Medium 3

Peptone	-	5 gm.
Yeast extract	-	1.5 gm.
Beef extract	-	1.5 gm.
Sodium Chloride	-	3.5 gm.
Glucose	-	1 gm.
Dipotassium Phosphate	-	3.68 gm.
Patassium Dihydrogen Phosphate	-	1.32 gm.
Distilled water To make up volume	-	1 litre.
pH After sterilisation	-	7.

Assay methods of different antibiotics mostly same only standard bacterial culture differ for different antibiotics assay.

Pollution Control

In the production by fermentation.

Efluent produce from antibiotics production centre by fermentation method content high B.O.D. and COD. level. It should be reduceby Bio-methanation technique. By this process produce methane gas can be used for fuel in the or boiler, Domestic uses.

Preservation Technique

Antibiotics produced by fermentation method or by chemical synthesis method are aseptically packed in sterile package which may be made by glass or special plastic container : All the antibiotics should be store below 15°C, preferebly below 4°c for keeping its proper activity.

Market

Table 1

Likely Demand of Potassium Penicillin-G and its derivatives Upto 2000 A.D.

SL. No.	Name	1984 -85	1989-90	Estimated 1994-95	Demand 1995-2000
I.	***Semi-synthetic penicillins (tonnes) :***				
1.	Ampicillins	286	580	1160	2300
2.	Amoxycillin	72	145	290	600
3.	Cloxacillin	19	30	55	100
4.	Others	-	5	10	20
	TOTAL (1)	379	760	1515	3020
II.	***Cephalosporins (tonnes) :***				
1.	Cephalexin	36	75	150	290
2.	Cephradine & others.	-	5	10	20
	TOTAL (II)	36	80	160	310

III. *Intermediates (tonnes) :*

(based on consumption norms)

1.	6-APA	230	460	918	1830
2.	7-ADCA	26	57	114	222
	TOTAL (III)	256	517	1032	2052

IV. *Potassium Penicillin-G (MMU) :*

(based on consumption norms)

1.	6-APA	713	1426	2846	5673
2.	7-ADCA	114	251	502	977
3.	Others	300	520	600	700
	TOTAL (IV)	1127	2197	3948	7350

V. *Demand for patassium penicillin - G(MMU) :*

1.	Intermediates	740	1850	3700	7400
2.	Formulations etc.	410	520		
	TOTAL (V)	1150	2370	3700	7400

Suppliers of Raw Materials :

1. Herdillia Chemicals Ltd.

   Air India Building

   Nariman Point.

   Bombay - 400021.

2. Catalysts and chemicals

   India Ltd.

   240, D. Nooroji Road,

   Bombay - 400001.

3. Calico chemicals Plastics and Fibres Division

   Anik-Chamber,

   Bombay - 400074.

4. Vasu Chemicals

   1-4 Geota Industrial Estate

   I.B. Patel Road,

   Goregaon (East)

   Post Box No - 9024,

   Bombay - 400063.

5. Hindustan Organic Chemicals Ltd.

   P.O. Rasayani,

   Dist. Kulaba

   Maharashtra.

6. The Dharamsi Moraji Chemical Company Ltd.

   Prospect chambers.

   317-321 Dr. D.N Road,

   Bombay - 400021.

7. International Solvent and Chemical Company,

   85, Nariman Bhawan

   Opposite Hoechst House,

   227, Nariman Point,

   Bombay - 400021

   Tel. : 2028162, 2024774

   Fax : 2040799.

8. A. Choksey Chemical Industries Ltd.

   101, M.G.Road,

Fort, Bombay - 400023,

Tel. : 273868, 274006,

Telex : 11-83716 PHOSIN.

9. Alpha Group (Hong Kong) Ltd.

Suite 1008,

Bank of America Tower,

Hong Kong.

Fax : 8525303830.

Tel. : 8525303800.

Telex : 71265 ALFA HX.

Plant and Machinery

Centrifuge, Fermentor, Reactor

1. M/s Vucan Ltd.

Mustafa Dupodi Building

7A, Sir P.M. Road.

Bombay - 400038.

2. Larsen and Toubro Ltd.

Landt House,

Powai,

Ballard Estate,

Bombay - 400038.

3. Dorr Oliver,

Hindustan Dorr-oliver Ltd.

Dorr-oliver House,

Chakala,

Andheri (east)

Bombay - 400099.

4. Buckau Wolf India Ltd,

Pimpri,

Pune - 411018

India,

Tel. - 84461.

Uses of Antibiotics

Amphotericins

Used as antifungal agents.

Chloramphenicol

A broad spectrum antibiotic which is effective against Gram-positive and Gramnegative bacteria and ricketetsia. It has been found to be particulary effective against salmonella typhosa and certain other salmonella species. It has produced very fovorable results in the treatment of typhus fevers which are caused by rickettsiae.

Cycloserine

It is broad specturm antibiotics. It is antibacterial agent. It has shown particular promise as an antitubercular agent.

Erythromycin

It is active against gram positive bacteria including micrococc, Strepto cocci, pneumococci, and corvnebacterium diphtheriae.

Neomycin

It is active against a large number of gramtive and gram-ve and acid-fast bacteria. It is a inactive against most yeasts, molds, protozoa and true viruses.

Because of its neurotoxicity nephrotoxicity and ability to produce permanent deafness, it's parenteral applications are limited.

Penicillin

It is active against certain gram positive bactria in the presence of blood, pus and body fluid

Streptomycin

It is effective against gram negative bactria, bactero statically, bacterio cidally, in vitro, and in the presence of body fluids and that would be relatively nontoxic to the cells and tissues of the body .

Tetracycline

They are widely used for conbating in fections in human being and animals including amoebiasis, diarrheas, shigellosis, and other disease condition.

Chlorotetracyline and Oxytetracycline are used in animal feeding, for the preservation of fooders and for other purposes.

Cost Anaslysis

(1)	Production	: 1 Ton/day = (1/6 M.M.U.)
(2)	Land and Built up area	: Rs.100,000,000
(3)	Plant and machinery	: Rs.80,000,000
(4)	Other fixed Cost	: Rs.20,000,000
(5)	Total fixed Capital Require	: Rs.200,000,000
(6)	Raw Matrial Require/3month	: Rs.32,500,000
(7)	Salary-wages/3months	: Rs.1,500,000
(8)	Other miscllaneous variable expenditure/3months	: Rs.6,000,000
(9)	Working Capital/3months	: Rs.40,000,000
(10)	T.C.I.	: Rs.240,000,000
(11)	Project Cost	: Rs.210,000,000
(12)	Production Cost/annum	: Rs.222,500,000
(13)	Sales Turnover/annum	: Rs.300,000,000
(14)	Profit per annum	: Rs.77,500,000
(15)	Profit Percent on T.C.I	: 32.29.%

(16) Profit Percent on Project Cost : 36.9%

(17) Fixed Cost/annum : Rs.126,500,000

(18) B.E.P. % : 62.0

3 BIOFERTILIZER

INTRODUCTION

Fertilizer a substance which helps to grow plants rapildly and produce fruits flower and vegetable more quantity in proper time, otherwise fetilizer be a compound, which fullfil the needed minerals orelemerts require for the growth of plants and vegetables to produce and products in proper time.

Fertilizer basically three types :

(1) Inorganic fertilizer (2) Organic ferrtlizer (3) Biofertilizer.

Biofertilizer are natural fertilizers which are inocrobial moculants of bacteria, algae, fungi alone or in combination and they augment the availability of nutrients to the plants. Rhizobium is the best known biofertilizer which fixes atmospher nitrogen symbiotically with legumes. Other bio-fertilizers are Azobacter, Azospirillum, Blue green algae and Azolla.

Biofertilizers actually counteract the toxic effects of chemical fertilizers in the soil. The use of biofertilizer, in preference to chemical fertilizers, offers economic and ecological benefits by way of soil health and fertility to fermers. Biofertilizers provide a dependable continued source of supply of nutrients unlike chemical fertilizers which, besides Cost, are depleting source and add upto the pollution problems.

The earliert production of Rhizobium in oculant in India started in 1934, but comercial production was undertaken in 1964 when soyabean

was introduced in the country subsequently there was increase in demand for bioferlilizers for other legumes also production of other biofertilizers such as Blue Gree Algae, Azotobacter, Azospirillum and Azolla is also undertaken in the country on large scale. There is a good demand for Azospirillum from farmers of Tamilnadu as they have obtained significant response in rice and sugar cane.

Although the bio-fertilizers cannot by themselves totally replace chemical fertilizers at least in the near future, there is need for integrated nutrient supply to crops through a judicious amalgam of biological, chemical and organic soirce of nutrient supply.

Among the different types of fertilizers available at present, Rhizobium is relatively more effective and more urdely used particularly the small and marginal farmers who constitute about 56% at the total farming community are reluctant to use chemical fertilizers in legumecultivation resulting in very poor yields. Considering the area cultivated under legume crop use of Rhizobium can be apromising input which can substantially increase legume crops.

Agriculture to-day Consumes high inputs of nitrogen. The present needs of nitrogen are largely met from synthetic nitrogen fertilizers their consumption has been rising every year. These fertilizers are quite expensive because of high cost of production consequently their high inputs have considerably increased agricultural production in a highly energy consuming process (13800 k cals per kg of nigrogen fixed). Therfore in the present situation of energy constraint, attention has diverted to tap alternatives to suppliment nitrogen resources by directly utilising atmosheric nitrogen through biological nitrogen through biological fixation. In the symbiotic nitrogen fixing system, photosynthctically stored cnergy is utiliscd instcad of fossil fuels. In this process atmospheric nitrogen is reduced to ammonia in presence of clectron donor (ferredoxin and flavodoxin), ATP. generating system and biological catalytser (nitrogenase, hydrogenase, and some minerals)

Manufacturing Process

Now symbiotic bacteria Azotobacter species has great role to fix atmospheric nitrogen in presence of carbohydrate or any other energy sourcess on that basis Azoto bacter agilis and Azotobacter chroococcum strain can be used for the production of biofertiliser.

Properly isolated pure suitable Azotobacter strain is stored at 4^{0}c in sterile and aseptic condition.

Took out Commercial usable Azotobacter agilis strain in a strile and aseptic condition. Transfer some spore by sterile platinumloop to a sterile test tube containing 10 ml, 2% molasses broth with 100 R.P.M. Phosphate ions keep the tests in the incubator for 5 days at 25°C. When the cells are properly growth then streatk some inocculam over sterile agar medium in ptridishes keep the ptridishes in the incubator at 25-30°C for 4-5 days, when the well seperated bacterial colony will be appeared, took minimum 15colonies from each ptridishes by sterile platinum loop and transfer it to the test tube (Containing 2%, 10ml sterile molasses with minerals), keep this test tube in the incubator at 25-30^{0}c for 2 days. After 2 days growth of bacteria in test tube trasfer to 3 litres conical flask containing 1 litre molasses media containing suitable minerals and pH greater than and less than 8% Ineabete The flaskin shaker at 30^{0}c with 30 R.P.M. for 4 days. Now this flask containing bacterial growth used for further aseptically transfer to 10 litre media of same composition in 20 litre vessels and keep it for 3 days at 25^{0}c which will be used at for commarcial inocculum.

Commercial Process

It can be produced by tray culture method or by submerge fermentation method.

In both cases proper aeration and agitation system required.

Media preparation

Took the weighted amount molasses in a steriliser, add water to it such that after steam strilization should be diluted to 2% wt by volume. Added to it 100 pp.m. Phosphate ions and 10 pp.m. boron, and znicions.

Sterile molasses transfer to fermentor or trays. Cool down the molasses temp at 25-30°C. Added to it 2% in oculum in the molasses medium at sterile condition. pH of the medium 6.5 - 7.5, Temp of the fermentation maintained 25° - 30°C. aeration rate 20% c.f.m. Time of fermentration 4-6 days. or time to fermented till the cells count more than 1 × 108 cells/ml.

When the required cells count atained, then this broth is mixed with carrier (peat or lignite or calcium carbonate) to moisture content 20-25%. carrier should be intially sterile and cool at 30°c. Carrier mixed with cells used for biotertiliser.

Carried mixed with the broth keep for 7 days to complete release of formed gasses and then it is packed by form fill and seal machine of about 200 gms per pack or more upto 5 kg/pack according to demand and market a or ailability. After poly packing it is again packed in corrugated cartoons and then marketed Biofertilizer should store at 25°c or below it. Activity of biofertiliser decrease or lost at 40°c.

It should be noted that there should be fermentation indefecient of nitrogen in theanedia and it should contains minerals micro amount of Boron, znic, cobolt and molybdebum which helper to growth of micro organism.

Test Parameters

(1) Green house test took the proper biofertilizers and dilufe to 500-1000 times and spray it on the soil or plants, the number of useful micro organism in the soil will increase. In presence of micro organism in creases the nitrogen quantity of the soil this fullfill the plants requirement of nitrogen partially or fully. By regular observation of plants growth confirm the effectiveness of biofetilizer.

(2) ***Cells count*** : Biofertiliser should content 10 millions active cells per gm. It should be checked by sterilamedia of bacto agar in ptridishes. It should also checked periodically upto six months.

Cells count microscopically : Took 1gm. sample or 1ml. sample in a test tube, add on it 5 ml distilled water and 1 ml of 1% methylene blue solution on it shake properly the test tube, put one drop of the sample in the hamecytometer slide from which calculate the total number of cells per ml. of the sanmple dead cells are absorb the blue colour, living cells are not absorb any colour.

(3) Gibson Tubetest

(4) Leonard Jar test

Pollution Control

Normally in case of biofertiliser plant, quantity of liquid efflient will be lower, washing of the plant will be the effluent. This effluent water is treated by lime solution to make it neutral and put in a reservoir tank or effluent water treated by bleaching powder and put in a reservoir. overflow of the treated effluent from 1st reservoir is aqrated by air and keep it store for 7 days before disposal.

Preservation Technique

Biofertiliser packed in polypack and store it in cool place at 25°C. or below that. Biofertiliser loss their activity at highei temperature. It will loss about complete it's activity at 40°C.

Again biofertiliser activity depend on the aeration, humidity of the soil and enviromental temp.

In a symbiotic process, certain nitrogen fixing bacteria grow in close association with higher plant, usually with its roots where nodulls are formed The process takes place in the nodulls throush enzyme system the nodules contain a soluble haemoglobin-type pigment namely, leghamoglobin, which facilitates oxygen uptake by terminal oxidase and increase A.T.P. production for nitrogenase activity. In the non-symbiotic process there is wide variaty of free living organism which fix atmosphric nitrogen under aerobic or an aerobic condition depending upon the organism and the conditions.

Market

There are more than 58 biofertilizer production units in the country with total production capacity of 2667 Tonnes per annum. Most of the production unit belong to the central Government, state government and agriculture universities and state government corporation, Private sector unit/share only 12.

Main manufacturers of biofertilisers are :

A. Gujrat state fertilizers Company Ltd.

P.O.- Fertiliser Nagar,

Dist : VADODARA

Pin : 391750.

This Company's brand name of biofertilizers "**SARDAR**"

They produces now 4 types of biofertiliser :

1. SARDAR Azotobacter culture :

   For the production of cereals, cash crops, and vegetables.

2. SARDAR Azospirillum culture :

   For cereals, cash crops and vegetables.

3. SARDAR Rhizobium culture :

   For the production of pulses, and legominos crops.

4. SARDAR Phosphate culture :

   Production for all crops.

B. NAFED.

C. Madras Fertiliser Limited.

It's brand name **Vijay** Biofertiliser.

D. Hindustan lever Research Centre

Andheri, Bombay,

Work on biofertiliser.

Response to Azospirillum inoculation in different crops :

Crop	Nitrogen applied kg/ha	No. of isolation	% increase over control
Rice	0	5	21.40
	40	-	10.50
Wheat	0	3	4.41
	40	-	13.80
Barley	0	6	16.70
	40	-	16.70
Oats	0	6	42.23
	40	-	17.44
Pearmillet	0	2	6.31

Estimated Potential of Biofertilizer in four Southern state:

(*Source Fertilizer News 1994*)

Name of the states	Estimated Production in Tons	Installed capacity in Tons
Andhra Pradesh	11382	175
Karnatak	8663	40
Kerela	517	--
Tamilnadu	5263	1100
Total	25825	1315

Fertilizer Import : (in million Tonns)

(Source Fertilizer News December 1994)

Year	Urea	DAP	MOB
1991-92	0.39	2.08	2.04
1992-93	1.86	1.53	1.96

It has no doubt that in future biofertilizer will take it's position over chemical synthetic fertilizer. Development of biofertilizer by application of genetic engineering technique will produce a biofertilizer which will stable at higher temperature , long self life and able produce crops higher amount whithin short period of time. It is undoubtedly we can predict that biofertilizer market demand will rapidly jump with the qwarness of farmers and self life increase.

Uses

In spite of many advantages use of biofertilizers in the country remained very low relative to the potential. tack of awareness among the farmers regarding the beneficial effects of the use of biofertilizer as well as it's availability are among the factors responsible for the low use.

BAIF has generated facilities to produce biofertilizers in fermentors specific to crops such as ground nut soyabean, moong, and bengal gram BAIF has undertaken studies to isolate and identify Rhizobium strains for selected multipurpose tree species (MPTS) which are suitable in agro-forestry and waste-land development programmes.

Biofertilizer used for the production rice, water, barley oats, sugarcane ground nuts. In future biofertilizer of different train of microbes will use for the cultivation of all the types of fruits, vegetables crops and cereals.

Azospirillum, a new nitrogen fixing associate symbiont, has shown promising results. It in creases yields of cereals amounting to a saving of fertilizer nitrogen equivalent to 20-40 kg N/ha.

10 kg soil containing 5% blue green algal per hectare is commercially used these days as a biofertilizer, amounting to saving of about 30 kg fertilizer nitrogen per hectore.

Suppliers of Raw Material :

Cell Culture

1. Tamilnadu Agriculture University, Coimbatore.
2. BAIF, Pune.
3. BATIELLE,

   505, King Avenue Columbus,

   Ohio 43201-2693

   USA.

   Tel. - 614/424-6424.

   Fax - 614/424-5263.
4. New Brumswick Scientific (U.K) Ltd.

   6,Colorial way,

   Watford, Herts,

   WD2 4PT

   Tel. - 0923-23293

   Tlx - 89418 BRUNCOG.
5. Haryana Agriculture University

   Hissar, HARYANA.

Chemicals/Biochemicals

6. Bio Business INDIA Ltd.

   C-76, Fateh Nagar,

   Jail Road,

   New Delhi - 110018

   INDIA.

   Tel. : 091-11-5596820
7. Biogentek B.G.

   C-10 Basement.

   Asoka Tower,

   C-Block Commercial Complex,

   Janakpuri,

   New Delhi - 110058.

   INDIA.

   Tel. - 091-11-5594620,

   5594917, 5508557

   Tlx : 031-65099 ABP IN.

   Fax : 011 -5555938.

Peat/lignite

1. Bharat Coaking Coal Ltd.

   Coal Bhawan

   Coal City

   Dhanbad.

2. United Carbon India Ltd.

   M.I.D.C. Plot No - 3

   Trans Thane creek Area

   Thane Belapur Road,

   Post : Ghansoli

   Thane - 400701

   Phone : 2021914 / 20278486 / 2027962.

Plant and Machinery Supplier :

Fermentors

1. Agram Industries

   126 Nelson Road,

   Aminjikarai,

   Madras - 600029

   INDIA.

   Tel. : 091 - 44 - 483543, 4838784.

   Tlx : 041-25030.

   Fax : 091-44 - 4835413.

2. Bio Business India Ltd.

   C-76, Fateh Nagar,

   Jail Road,

   New Delhi - 110018

   INDIA.

   Tel. : 091-11-5596820

   Tlx : 031-61922

   Fax : 091-11 - 5596820.

3. Alfa Laval (India) Limited.

   Dapodi, Pune - 411012.

   Tel. : 82321 (6 lines)

Sealing Machine

1. Vibgyor International Pvt. Ltd.

   904 Pragati Tower,

   26 Rajendera Palace

   New Delhi - 110008

   Tel. : 5711757, 5718363.

2. Crystal Engineering Co India.

   WZ - 2C/1 Basai Darbar,

   Near Shiv Mandir

   (Behind Natraj Cinema)

   New Delhi - 110015.

   Tel. : 591628.

Mixing Machine

1. Samarpan Fabricator Ltd.
   Plot No. A-182 / A-183.

   Lane-Z, Room No-16,

   Wagle Industrial Estate

   Thane - 400604.

   Tel. : 505373 / 505630 / 505653.

Laboratory Analytical Instrument

1. Chemtron Analytical Instruments (P) Ltd.

   306, 9/2 East Patel Nagar,

   New Delhi - 110008.

   INDIA.

   Tel. - 091-11 - 5755987,

   Fax - 091-11-5724135.

2. Sartoriws Biotech (India) Pvt. Ltd.
   812, Barton Centre.

   84, M.G. Road.

   Bangalore - 560001

   INDIA.

   Tel.: 09-80-3303040, 3302655
   Tlx : 845-2999.

   Fax : 091-80 - 5882392.

3. Biogentek BG.

   C-10 Basement,

   Ashoka Tower,

   C-Block, Commercial Complex

   Janakpuri,

   New Delhi - 110058.

   INDIA.

   Tel. : 09-11 - 5594620, 5594917

   Tlx : 031-65099 ABPIN.

   Fax : 011- 5555938.

4. LEICA Microscopy & System GmBH

   Postfach - 2040

   D-35530, Wetzlar

   Germany.

   Tel. : (06441) 29-0

   Tlx : 0041 - 483849.

   Fax : (06441) 293399 and 2339.

Biofertilizer

1.		Production capacity	:	10T/day
2.	(a)	Land Required 5000 sqm.		
		Rate Rs. 500/sqm.	:	Rs.2500000
	(b)	Built up Area - 1000sqm.	:	Rs20,00000
		Rate 2000/s		
	(c)	Land develop area	:	Rs.500000
3.		Plant and Machinery	:	Rs.50,00000
4.		Other fixed Cost	:	Rs.10,00000
5.		Fixed Capital required	:	Rs.1,10,00000
6.		Raw Material	:	Rs.15,000
7.		Salary / wages / month	:	Rs.200000
8.		Other Revenue expenditure /Month	:	Rs.100000
9.		W/C for 3 month	:	Rs.11,25,000
				Rs.6,00000
				Rs.3,00000
				Rs.20,25,000

10.	T.C.I	:	Rs.1,10,00000
		Add	Rs.20,25 000
			Rs.1,30,25,000
11.	Project Cost	:	Rs.11,000,000
		Add	Rs.506,250
			Rs.11,506,250
12.	Production Cost /annum	:	Rs.11,653,750
13.	Sales Turnover / annum		
	10,000 × 300 × 6	:	Rs.18,000,000
14.	Profit per annum	:	Rs.6,346,250
15.	Fixed Cost	:	Rs.6,793,750
16.	Break Even Point (B.E.P.)	:	51.70%

4 INSULIN AND GROWTH HORMONE

Introduction

Genetic Engineering offers an alternative approach to the pharmacuatical industry and human hormos can now be produced by genetically manipulated bacteria. The marketing of insulin and growth hormone obtained by genetic engineering techniques has already been authorised in numerous country. In France the human growth hormon represents the first therapeutical substance to produced in large scale in bacteria. The production is carried out in industrial fermentors by the pharmaceutical compacy Sanafe. Willem Roskam explain why studies on the human growth hormone cancern the entire parmacuitical industry, not only an account of the hormone itself, but also because the entire new technology develop to produce it represent a model for the manufacture of other proteins of therapeutical interest. to bring the benefit arising from such chemical and biological research to general public it was also necessary to improve industrial production technique. This entailed firstly the ability to synthesize the therapentical substance on a large scale, Secondly it was indispensible to veryfy that the industrial procedure always gave the desired molecule. Thirdly the level of residual Contaminated formed during the synthesis had to be well below the level at which side effects might be observed.

To treat some diseases doctors need to use complex molecules, for example protein extracted from animal or human tissues. These proteins can be either hormones such as insulinor enzymes, such as factor VIII. Insulin used to treat diabetics in extracted from the pancreas of pigs or oxen obtained directly from slaughtter house. Factor VIII, Which plays a part in blood coagulation is used to treat patients lacking this factor

and suffering from haemophilia. Factor VIII is extracted and concentrated from human plasma.

In fact since the turn of 1980's industrial genetic engineering has developed to the extent that processes have been devised for producing diversity of proteins such as insulin growth hormone,tissue plasminogen activator (an enzyme involve in the dissolving of clots which obstract the artiries) interleukin -2 (a substance involved in the activition of certain cells of the immune system), interferon (on antiviral substanec) etc.

However the utilisation of proteins for theraplutic purpose, presents some limitations. In general they cannot be administered orally as they are usually destroyed in the digestive tube. They Have to be injected inter venously or, intramas cularly.

The biotechnology industry cut its teeth making pharmaceutical proteins with genetically engineered bacteria. But it is moving on to more sophisticated production system using mammalian cell culturs instead of micro organism.

Beyond that, researchers expect soon to be able to extract human proteins from the milk of a transgenic farm animals and perhapes also from plants. In the long run, the cheapest way of producing some pharmacuticals could be as an agricultural crop.

When the first biopharmaceutical Companies started up in the late 1970's scientists hand only recently invented the recombinant DNA technology which makes it possible to transfer a gene from one species to another, They begen working with the simplest and best understood system, the bacterium E. Coli and quickly Scaled up the process so that bacterial cultures could make large quantities of human proteins. The first genetically engineered drug was human insulin, originally developed by Genetech in the U.S and launefed by Eli lilley in 1982.

Manufacturing Process of Insulin

(a) Industrial production of insulin by using genetically manipulated bacteria E. Coli of special strain.

(b) Insulin canbe prepared from the pancrease of pigs or oxen obtained directly from slaughter house.

Manufacturing Process of Insulin and growth Hermone

These can be produced from the especially developed genetically Engineered special strain of Escheriachia coli by Submerge fermentation method.

Following media Compositon used for chemostat growth of Escherichia coli.

Component		Concentration Per litre
Glucose	-	5gm.
KH_2PO_4	-	3gm.
K_2HPO_4	-	7gm.
$(NH_4)_2SO_4$	-	1gm.
$MgSO_4$,$7H_2O$	-	0.492gm.
Trace Mineral Solution	-	1ml.
Vitamins Solution	-	1ml.

Cells are grown at specific growth rate from $0.04h^{-1}$ to $0.25h^{-1}$ at 30°c. It has been found that acetate accumulation starts at the speaific growth rate 0.14h in^{-1} the growth media.

Component of culture media

Water -Good quality water should be free from all the ions, bacteria and organic molecules i.e water used should be sterile water should store in container such that there is no metal should be leached out.

Water should be tested regularly for conductivity, presence of organics and presence of pyrogens from contaminating organism.

Basal Media

Most cell culture media contain a mixture of salts, vitamins, aminoacids, Co-enzymes and minerals generally called basal medium.

Most cell culture media use sodium bicarbonate as the pH buffering system.

Aminoacids in Busal Media are : Arginine, cysteine, half cysteine Glutamin, histidine, Isolusine, lucine lysine etc.

Sugar Neucleic Acids and intermediaats in Basal Media : Glucose plyvuvate acetate, ribose, deoxyriboseHypoxanthine, Xanthine, Thymine, thymidine, uracil.

Lipids and Derivatives

Cholesterol, choline, ionositol, Linoleic acid.

Vitamins and Coenzymes in Basal media : Ascorbic acid, Biotine, Folicacid, p-amino Benzoic acid, α lipoic acid, Nicotinic Acid etc.

Inorganic Ions in basal Media : Calcium, Magnesum, Potasium, Sodium, Chloride, Phosphorus, Sulfate and Nitrate.

Trace elements : Iron, cobalt, Copper, (Cu) Zinc.

The fermentation may be carried out at temperature 30°c and pH-7.0. Approximately 7.5 Hrs after inocculation the glucose level dropped to less than 2 gm/litre at which point the feed of the nutrient solution should start. Feed rate of the nutrient solution sould be such that specific growth rate of the cells will' be between 0.1 - 0.14h^{-1}. This can be maintained by addition of feed at the rate of 1ml per gram of cell dry weight per hour. It is observe that acetate concentration. should not increase 0.5gm/litre.

Aerationrate 2 V.V.M and agitation 60-70 R.P.M.

Following Media Composition used for the high cell density growth of E Scherchia coli.

Component	Batch Media Concentration Per litre 5gm	Feed Media Concentration 433gm Per litre.
Glucose	5gm	433gm
Yeast Extract	5gm	--
K_2HPO_4	7gm	--
KH_2PO_4	8gm	1gm
$(NH_4)_2SO_4$	5gm	105gm
Mg SO_4, $7H_2o$	1gm	8.5gm
Trace Mineral Solution	2 ml	56 ml
Vitamin Solution	2 ml	56 ml
Ampicilin	0.5gm/lr.	--

Initial inocculum cells density will be 1.5 x 10^6 cells/ml and final cells density will be 1.5 -2 x 10^8 cells/ml/ when cells concentration will transfer to commercial fermentor or seprate the cells from the fermented broth.

Cells and fermented broths are seperated and then further process to Seperate the end products. After getting end product, again the product is pass through the purification process. Purified products are collected in properly cleaned microbe free Container. Store at 40°C or below that temperature.

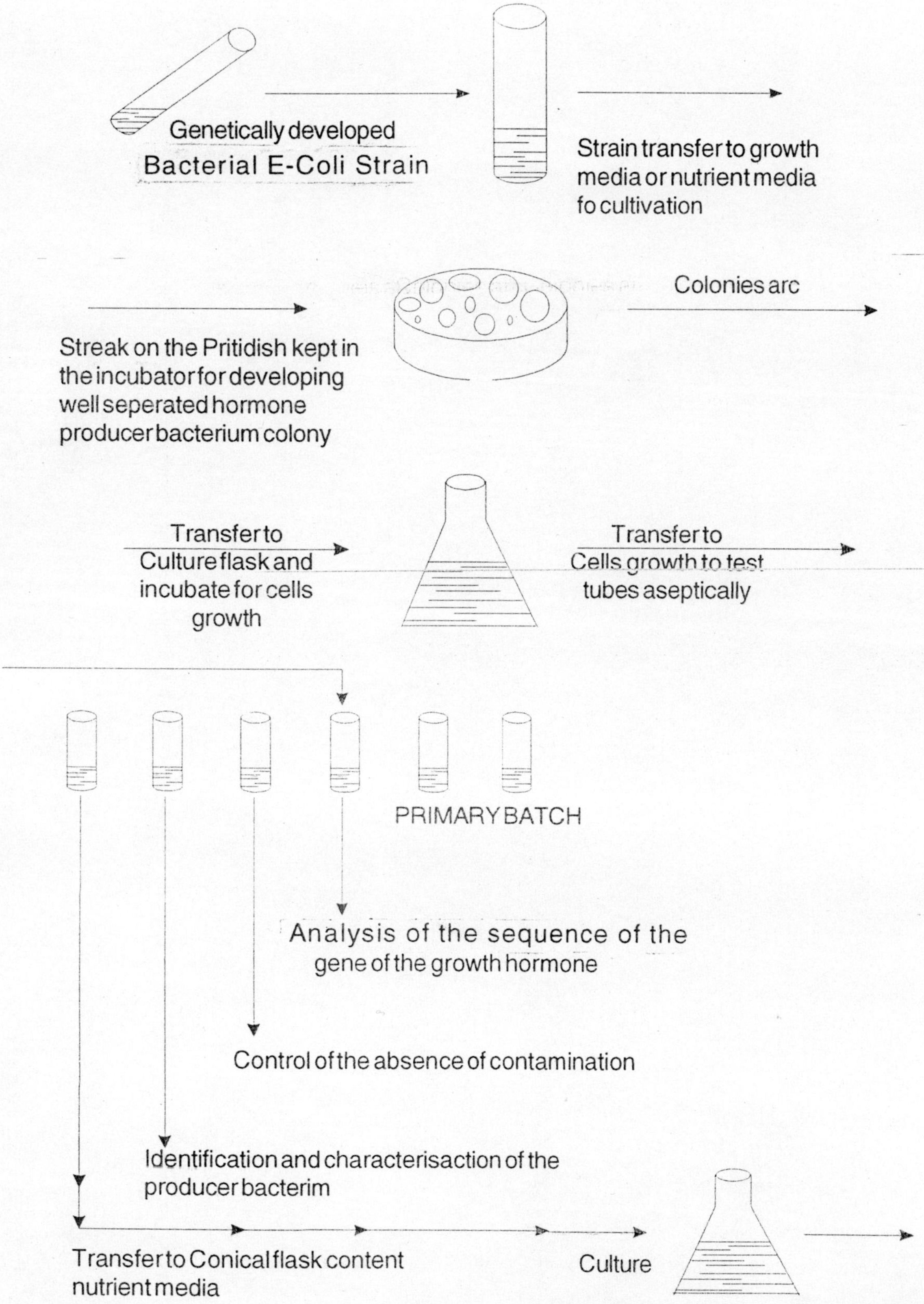
Genetically developed
Bacterial E-Coli Strain
Strain transfer to growth media or nutrient media fo cultivation
Streak on the Pritidish kept in the incubator for developing well seperated hormone producer bacterium colony
Colonies arc
Transfer to Culture flask and incubate for cells growth
Transfer to Cells growth to test tubes aseptically
PRIMARY BATCH
Analysis of the sequence of the gene of the growth hormone
Control of the absence of contamination
Identification and characterisaction of the producer bacterim
Transfer to Conical flask content nutrient media
Culture

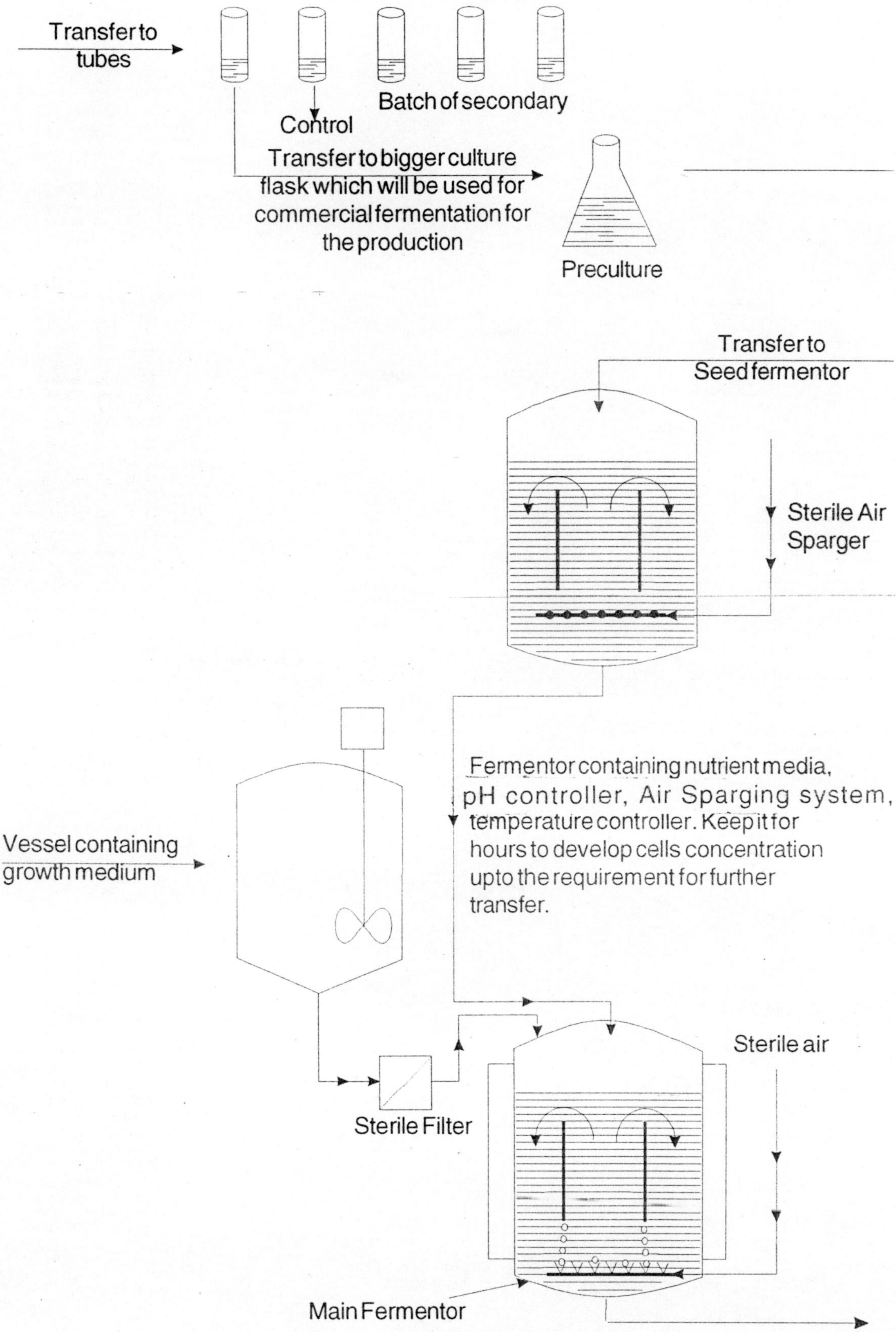
Transfer to tubes
Batch of secondary
Control
Transfer to bigger culture flask which will be used for commercial fermentation for the production
Preculture
Transfer to Seed fermentor
Sterile Air Sparger
Fermentor containing nutrient media, pH controller, Air Sparging system, temperature controller. Keep it for hours to develop cells concentration upto the requirement for further transfer.
Vessel containing growth medium
Sterile Filter
Sterile air
Main Fermentor

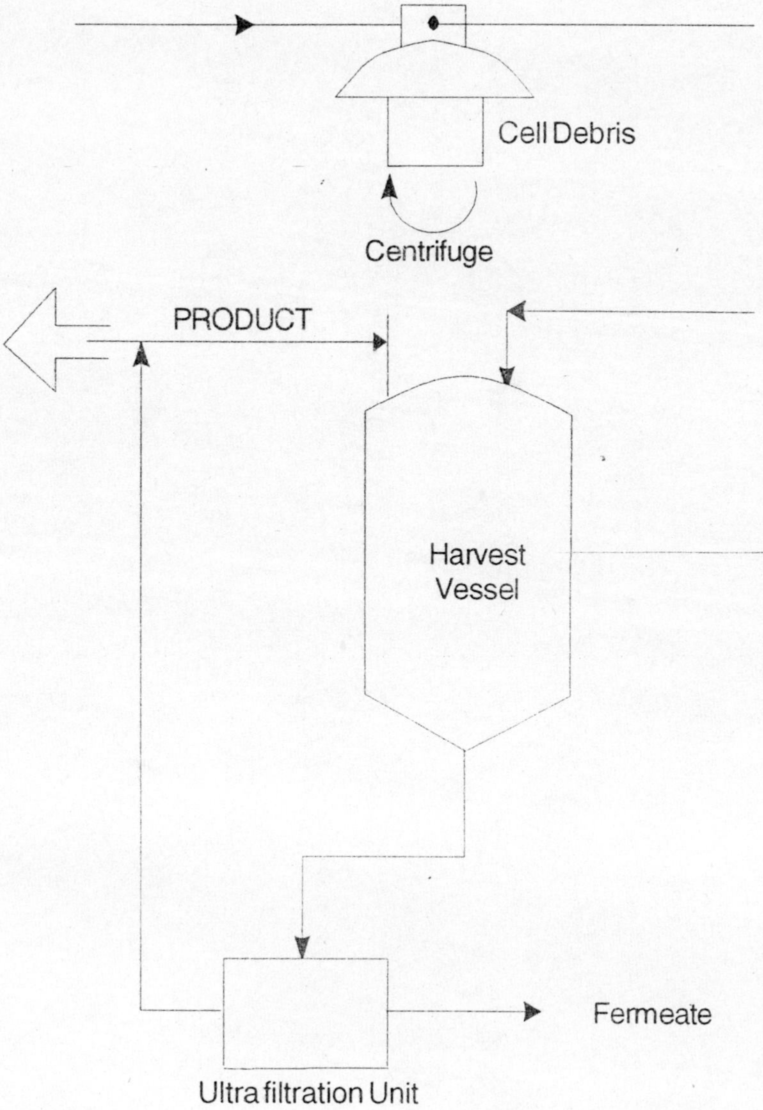
Cell Debris
Centrifuge
PRODUCT
Harvest
Vessel
Fermeate
Ultra filtration Unit

Plant Machinery Suppliers

Lab equipment

1. *Microbalanes*

The Sientcfic instrument Co. Ltd.
A-15, Mohan Co-operative
Industrial Estate,

Mathura Road,

New Delhi - 110044

India

Tel. : 091-11-6849187, 634260.

Tlx : 031-75446 Sico in

Fax : 091-11-687476.

2. *Aseptic Environ Systems*

(a) Heraeus Instrument G.M.BH

Indian Representative office :

411, International Trade
Tower, Nehru Place,

New Delhi - 110019

INDIA.

Tel. : 091-11-6424038,
6469568

Fax : 091-11-6466721

(b) Klenzaids Bioclean Devices (P) Ltd.

A-21 M.I.D.C.

Street No. 3

Andheri (East)

Bombay - 400093

India.

(c) Yorco Sales Private Ltd.

11 Netaji Subhas Marg

Darya Ganj,

New Delhi - 110002

India.

Tel. : 091-11-3278381,
3278306

Tlx : 031-65354 YORK IN.

Fax : 091-11-3264042.

3. *Autoclaves*

(a) Analytical Supplies Ltd.

Duffeld Road,

Little Eaton, Derby

DE25DR

Tel. : 0332831671

Tlx : 37405.

(b) Astell Seientific

172 Brown hill Road

London SE 62 DL

Tel. : 01-697-8811

Tlx : 8951810.

(c) Yorco Sales Private Ltd.

11, Netaji Subash Marg,

Daryaganj,

New Delhi - 110002.

India.

Tel. : 091-11-3278381

3278306

Tlx.: 031 - 65354 York in

Fax : 091 - 11 - 3264042

4. *H.P.L.C.*

(a) Bio Pad Pacific Ltd.

C-248, Defence Colony,

New Delhi - 110024

India

Tel. : 091 - 11 - 4610103

Fax : 091 - 11 - 4610765

(b) Blue Star Ltd.

SAHAS 414/2,

Veer Savarkar Marg.

Prabhadevi,

Bombay - 400025

India.

Tel. : 091-22-4306155

Tlx : 011-71193.

Fax : 091-22-4307078.

5. ***Micro Scope***

CARL ZEISS

Post fatch : 1380, D-7082

Oberkochen

Germany.

Tel. : 00497364203970

Tlx : 41-7135155

Fax : 0049736202382

(Agent India)

TOSHNIWAL BROTHERS

(Bombay) PVT. LTD.

198, Jamshedji Tata Road,

Bombay - 400020, India

Tel. : 091-22-22-1565, 221546

Tlx : 022-84123 JBPL

Fax : 091-22-2040396.

Commercial Equipment

1. Fermentors

(a) Toshniwal Brothers (P) Ltd.

Hemkunt House,

Flat No. 808

6, Rajendra Place,

New Delhi - 110008

(b) Buckau Wolf India Ltd,

Pimpri,

Pune - 411018

India.

Tel. - 84461

(c) Bennet and Company Ltd.

P.O. Box - 46

Andover, Hampshire

Tel. : 0980 - 64488.

(d) αH Fermentation Limited.

Bells Hill,

Stoke Poges,

Bucks

SL 24EG.

Tel. : 02814 - 5100.

Tlx. : 848296 α HFRM.

2. Centrifuge

(a) Precision Analytical

Instruments Pvt Ltd,

3-B, Pusa Road,

New Delhi - 110005

India.

Tel. : 091-11-5738169

Tlx : 031-77078

Fax : 091-11 - 5754489,

(b) Alfa Laval (India) Ltd.

Dapodi, Pune - 411052,

Tel. No : 82321 (6 lines)

3. Ultra filter Unit

(a) Filtech Pharma Lab Pvt Ltd,

Star Metal Compound.

L.B.S. Marg.

Vikhroli (West)

Bombay - 400083.

India.

Tel. : 091- 22 - 57825591
(563)

(b) Millipore (India) Pvt. Ltd.

50-A, 2nd Phase,

Ring Road,

Peenya, Bangalore.

Pin : 560058

India.

Tel. : 091 - 80 - 8396320.

Tlx : 0845 - 5089 MLPRIN

Fax : 091 - 80 - 8396345.

4. Air Filter

(a) Klenzaids Bioclean Devices (P) Ltd.

A - 21 M.I.DC,

Street No - 3

Andheri East,

Bombay - 400093

INDIA.

5. ULTRA LOW TEMPERATURE FREEZER : 86°C to - 152°C

(a) ASR Instruments

Baba Chambers,

73 Richmond Road,

Bangalore - 560025,

India.

Tel. : 091- 802212748,
12213196

Fax : 091 - 80 - 5583539.

(A) Raw Material Suppliers

Pharmaceuticals Media and Cellculater

(1) Genetix

C - 88 Kirti Nagar,

New Delhi - 110015

India.

Tel. : 091-11-5421714,
5467637

Tlx : 031 - 72121

Fax : 091 - 11 - 5467637.

(2) Pharmacia Biotech Far East Ltd.

A - 3 Palani Towers,

31 Venkat Narayan Road,

T.Nagar, Madras - 600017,

India.

Tel. : 091 - 44 - 4340747,
4346570.

Tlx : 041 - 23260

Fax : 091 - 44 - 434537

(B) Fine Chemicals :

(a) Bio Business India Ltd.

C - 76, Fateh Nagar,

Jail Road,

New Delhi - 110018

India.

Tel. : 091 - 11 - 5596820

Tlx : 031 - 61922

Ref : Biotechnology - Editor; J Rahim and G.Read; Volume 7b.

G.R. Jacobsen and S.O. Joky.

Properties of Insulin

Molecular wt about 6000- All crystal insulin preparation contain small amounts of heavy metals such as Zinc, Nickel, Cobalt or Cadmium. These are not impuritier, but normal Components of the molecule. Crytals, hexagonal System, usually obtained as flat rhombo hedra containing 0.4% Znic. Readily Soluble in dilute acids and alkalis but practically insoluble from pH 4.5 - 7.0

Isoelectric point 5.30 - 5.35.

In Considering the suitability of the expression system utilized to produce insulin (or any other biological product for that matters). The overriding consideration is the biological activity of the recombinant product for insulin E.Coli has been satisfoetory host cell. Many Properties of recombinant derived insulin have been essentially indistinguishable from those of porcine derived insulin including (1) Receptor binding invitro (2) Biological response invitro in isolated cells such as adipocytes, lymphocytes and fibroblasts (3) Blood glucose lowering and (4) Plasma Insulin pharma cheutical.

Human derived Insulin is absorbed from infection sites slightly rapidly then protien derived Insulin.

Human Growth Harmone

The products of genetically engineered bacteria are not always identical to the natural molecules in the human body. These differences are because bacteria can only make simple unadorned protein molecules while human and other mammalian cells frequently add other chemical chains to the basic protein.

The most abundant molecule has a molecular weight of around 22000 and even if used entirely alone. The protein consist of a chain of 191 amino acids the formula being establishes in 1969, notable by the team headed by C.H.Li in the United States. The amino acids chain is folded in space and its configuration is kept stable by two disulphide bridge fromed between some sulphur atom carried by certain amino acids of the chain.

Uses

Human Growth Harmone

It is used as injectable to keep balanced growth of the human. A total lack of growth harmone leads to dwarfism.

For example the normal height of the six year old child is 1.10 meter. A child of this age who is partially different in the growth harmone will only attain a height of 0.90 meter, which is that of a 4 year old. A total lack of growth hormone leads to dwarfism. The height of the individual will not exceed one meter on maturity.

Insulin

It is used as injectable for the treatment of diabetics.

Preservation of Insulin and human

It should be preserved ultra low temperature freezer *i.e.*, temperature below - 86°C for long storage.

Pollution Control

After centrifugation waste liquid effluent which comes out from insulin industries contents high B.O.D. and C.O.D. value. For reduce the B.O.D. and C.O.D. lead from effluent it is require to treat water effluent by three stages.

(*a*) Anerobic treatment

(*b*) Aerobic treatment

(*c*) lastly pisiculture treatment.

Anerobic Treatment

Produce effluent is passed through the tower type reactor content seeds (Produced from cow dung). Recirculate the effluent through reactor in close circuit at pH 6.5 - 7.5 temp 30° - 40°C. Initially recirculation continued around 15 - 20 days, such that pH should not decrease if pH decrease, make pH balanced by addition of lime solution. In the anerobic process methane gas produced and use it for domestic purpose or boiler purpose. By this process B.O.D./C.O.D. value of the effluent is reduced to 60% - 80%.

Aerobic Treatment

When the B.O.D./C.O.D. value is reduced to 60% - 80%, then effluent is passed through aerobic treatment. By aerobisis again B.O.D./ C.O.D. value will be come down to 80% - 90%.

Pisi culture Process

Balance 10 - 20% B.O.D./C.O.D. value is effluent will be further comes down to 95% by cultivation fish in the effluent. When the residual value of B.O.D./C.O.D. will remains, it can be throughout the ground as it is or by diluting it with water.

Market Studies

There is tremendous growth of World Market and Indian Market of human growth harmone and insulin. Both the above products are daily needed medicine.

Biotechnology, Strong Commercial future

Product	Sales in 1988 ($ million)
Insulin	150
Growth Harmone	150
Alpha Interferon	80
TPA	170
Hepatitis B vaccine	100
Total	650

By this year (1995), Biotechnology based products sales reach to $4000 million or 3 % of the world market.

Anticancer

Product	Sales ($ million)
Interferons	350
Interleukins	250
Immuno Conjugates	350
Mono Colonals against	
Septic Stock	300
E.P.O.	950
Colony Stimulating factor	275
Human Growth Harmones	250
Vaccines	300
Thrombolytics	350
Insulin	550
Total	3925

Cost Analysis

1)	Production	1 MU Insulin/day
2)	Land and Built up Area	Rs.7,50,00,000
3)	Plant and Machinery	Rs.5,24,00,000
4)	Other fixed Cost	Rs.1,93,00,000
5)	Total fixed Cost	Rs.14,67,00,000
6)	Raw Materials Required per 3 months	Rs.1,01,25,000
7)	Salary and wages per month	Rs.2,60,000
8)	Other 3 months variable expenditure	Rs.57,45,000
9)	Working Capital Required per 3 month	Rs.1,66,50,000
10)	Total Capital Investment	Rs.16,33,50,000
11)	Project Cost	Rs.15,08,62,500
12)	Production Cost/annum	Rs.10,74,22,500
13)	Sales Turnover/annum	Rs.15,00,00,000
14)	Profit/annum	Rs.4,25,77,500
15)	Profit percent on T.C.I.	26.06%

16) Profit percent on project cost	28.22%
17) Fixed Cost	Rs.6,74,62,500
18) B.E.P.	61.3%

5 AQUA CULTURE

Introduction

Biotechnology is an emerging technology with great potential. The country has the necessary talent to harness the potential of this technology. Technical innovation and resulting chnages is the key to the process of economic development . Determining the choice of future technologies thus becomes important economic priority for the nation. Today we are living in a society which is witnessing results of Technological development at such unprecented rate which could not have been imagined even 50 years back.

Biotechnology the technological gap between advanced nations and to the development country. Biotechnology, defined in a broad sense, is the application of biotechnological organism and molecules to technical and industrial processes. The fermentation process which were first established after the 2nd world war were used to produce new products such as steroid, antibiotics, and fine chemicals. And the biotechnology arises from a wave of innovation occuring within this fermentation process and results from application of different techniques. It generally implies the application of novel microbes and other living system, altered or modified through various technologies like genetic engineering, Biotechnological tools enable us to manipulate the core of all living matters i.e the DNA is a manner resulting in enhanced or even totally new properties in plants animals and micro organisms, thus providing vast scope for application in many areas like accelerated food production disease control, environment protection and improvment etc. In other words , its application are multisectorol.

Potential application area of biotechnology are

1. Agriculture

a) Biofertilizers

b) Bioinsecticide and Bio-pesticides

c) Hybrid seeds

d) Artificial seeds

e) Photosynthesis improvers

f) Stress Resistant crops and plants

g) Tissue culture

2. Animal husbandary

3. Aquaculture

4. Therman Health

a) Vaccines

b) Immunodiognistics

c) Medicines

5. Population Control

6. Fuel and fodder

7. Biomass from various sources

8. Waste

9. Chemical Feedstock.

Aquaculture Techniques

With 7000Kms of coastline and 4.5 million hectares of water area as ponds, tanks and lakes, aquaculture potential of India is yet to be harnessed fully. The potential areas of application of biotechnology in Indian fresh water aquaculture are recycling of organic matter, biological nitrogen fixation and genetic transfers. For example, average yield per hectare per annum of prawns in countries like Thailand, Phillippines, Taiwan, Hong Kong etc. is 10-12 tonnes compared to 300-400 tones in India. Above levels of high yields is possible by systamatic use of marine biology and pisciculture knowledge.

Various biotechnological tools are being utilized for use in aquaculture for improving productivity both in terms of quantity and quality or for providing value added products.

Production Techniques

It is estimated that India has a brackish water area of 11.90 lakh hectares. The major centers of brackish water prawn farming lying in the coastal regions of maritime states of India. At present the land used for brackish water aquaculture is limited to 82000 hectares from where only 62000 tonnes of prawn are produced.The rest of the area is idle or unutilised.

Site selection

Detailed engineering investigation has to be carried out to collect sufficient field data comprising of soil condition,water availability,topographical features, position of creeks canals,availability of power and road links. Marigrove land should not be used for culture and should be allowed for natural growth which helps for soil binding and nutrient cycling. Similarly agricultural land also should not be selected for brackish water shrimp culture.Only marginal land not used for agriculture should be used for brackish water shrimp farming. After detailed site survey topographic maps are prepared which are essential for planning layout of the farm.Information on total height of the region and levelling of ground are very important.Subsoil investigation are necessary to obtain engineering properties of soil which are required for designing the foundation of various farms structures.Testing of permiability of the soil is very important to measure the rate at which water seeps vertically.After completion of engineering investigation the data is used to prepare hydrographic and soil profile plan.Shrimp farm layout when properly designed should strike a balance considering economy,functionality and aesthetics.The basic principle is to minimise the number of gates,the sizes and length of dikes and canals but it should not sacrifice biological requirements of suitable enviornment of the culture species.The shrimp farms are designed as farmted system which suits for semintensive culture practices.

Pond Preparation

Pond preparation is the start of the culture operation and involves planning and coordination of schedules to maximise resources without compromising basic principles of shrimp production.The pond should be prepared at least 30-45 days prior to water culture.This is important to allow physical disintegration and chemical decomposition of minerals and organic matters from soil and adjust pH to slightly alkaline(7-8).

Non Acidic Sulphate Soil

The non acidic sulphate soil has pH value of more than 6.The soil is recognised by a dark to light brown colour and a clay to sandy clay texture.

Acidic Sulphate Soil

Acidic sulphate soil has very less pH(3-4).The soil is recognizable by the raddish colour (of iron oxide) that may form on the pond bottom after flooding.In the process concentration of iron and aluminium,which one harmful to the shrimp are released from soil.

Pond preparation for recloiming acid sulphate soil to pH above 5 includes steps such as (a) drying,cultivating and submerging and (b) refilling,flushing and liming.In case where a thin layer of non acid top soil overlay soil materials with high potential acidity,it may be advisable to excarate the pond bottom to a desired depth and fill back with non acid top soil.

Components Of Farm

The various farm components are reservoir system of ponds comprising nursery,rearing ponds, bioponds, supply canal, dikes, water control stuctures, pumps and supporting facilities like buildings, pump house, storage sheds and roads.

Pond

Before pond layout is planned it is necessary to keep in mind the requirement of size and shape of ponds such as pre growing pond, rearing pond and bio-pond. While desiging the farm a minimum space of 500m (buffer zone) between adajecnt farms and drinking water source should be maintained.

Pre-growing Pond

Pre-growing pond are nursery pond used for rearing fry up PL 20 stage after which they are transfered to rearing ponds. Pre growing pond will be in 10% of the total production area,shape will be square or rectangular. Pre growing ponds can be detected if PL 20 seeds are obtained from hatchey.

Rearing Ponds

It is used for growing from PL 20 to marketable size at the harvest stage. It's size will be 70% of the total production area, it's shape will be rectangular of the length and breadth ratio 1.15:1. Sometimes the shape of the ponds depends on the shape of site. The size of the grow out pond range from 1ha to 10ha. But for management convenience ponds beyond 5ha is not preferred.Bottom should be free from projected rocks, tree stumps etc.The pond bottom must have a gradual slope (3/1000) from the inlet gate towards drainage gate.

Bio Ponds

It is for satisfaction of pollution control authorities and to prevent environment degradation, drainage water from the farm should be acceptable to flow to the area or river system or sea. Bio ponds are necessary as part of the culture pond system. Bio ponds are large setting where the rich nutritional affulent are treated naturally. Bio ponds are also used for culture of fish, mussel etc. Bio ponds constitute about 7-10% of the total farm area.

Dike

The entire farm is provided with dikes or bands.there are three types of dike:-

1. Main dike, 2. Secondary dike, 3. tirtiary dikes.

1. ***Main dike*** is to protect the prawn farm from destruction due to flood, storm and tide etc.

2. Secondary Dike

Smaller in size to the main peripheral dike, they are usually provided on both sides of the main supply or drainage canal of and secondary supply or drainage canal. The total height is obtained by providing suitable free board of 0.3m. The top secondary dike is usually 1.5m and side slopes 1:1.5.

3. Tertiary Dike

Tertiary dikes are constructed between ponds. They should be able to contain the desired depth of water in the pond. The total slope of the top will be fixed in the same manner as the secondary dike.

Water Control Structure

The water flow in the pond system are controlled by various control structures which are (i) Main supply gate of farm, (ii) secondary supply canal control gate, (iii) Supply canal drain gate, (iv) Pond inlet gate, (v) Pond outlet gate and (vi) Farm main drainage gate.

Pumping station

Calculation of pump capacity requirement will be based on parameters such as pond area, average water depth in ponds, duration of pumping, water exchanges and efficiency of the pump. Pumping requirement of farm are of high capacity and low head type.

Outlet Gate Screen

The most size of the screen is related to average body weight (ABW) of the prawn. For prawn weight ranging from 0.5gms to 15gms, mesh size varies from 0.5mm to 10mm at the entrance gate. Screen is necessary to prevent loss of culture prawn.

Flushing

Flush is performed immediate after harvest of the pond. For preparing the pond, the bottom soil of the pond has to be ploughed. It overturn the wet soil and oxidize throughly.

Liming

When the pH of the water is above than 6.5, there is HO requirement of liming. When the pH is below 6, $CaCO_3$ or $Ca(OH)_2$ may be used according to requirements.

Table I : Lime Requirement In Relation To pH

pH	$CaCo_3$ Kg/ha	$Ca(OH)_2$ Kg/ha
4.0	1610	1070
4.5	1430	915
5.0	1050	672
5.5	720	460
6.0	340	217
6.5and above	0	0

Water Culture

This is done after pond preparation with the objective of establishing plytoplankton and zooplankton population at proper densities by filling the pond with properly screened brackish water which is conditioned and fertilised with organic and inorganic fertiliser.

Availability Of The Prawn Seeds

The brackish water adajecent to coasts, back waters, narigroves, estuaries and the surf area are known to be good grounds of collecting prawn seeds.

In case of a large scale production system of prawn should collect appropriate seeds from hatchery.

Hatchery

The process involves demonstration of external appearance of various stages of ovary development to fishermen/collection to enable them to arrive at the correct selection of quality broodstock,transport techniques of the animals,acclimatisation and proper stocking procedure into the maturation/spawning tank of the hatchery.

Maturation

Inside the maturation tank broodstock are given appropriate feed of excellent quality under semi controlled enviornment with proper water management,feeding and breeding practices,the female become gravid and ready for spawning.

Spawning

The gravid females are selected and transfered into spawning tanks with semi controlled condition to allow spawing to take place over night. Immediately after spawning eggs are analysed with regard to quality and quantity. Eggs are also washed and prepared for hatching into larvas.

Stages Of Larva

There are four stages : (a) Nauplius (b) Protozoea (c) Mysis and (d) Post Larva(PL).

In larva stages temperature maintained is 20°C for 35 - 40 hrs.

Feed in the larva stages (1) Planktonic food produced by using chemical fertilizer or diatom bloom or soyabean waste.

After 4 days protozoea become mysis stage.

Mysis stage last for 3 days at 28°C and passes to post larvae(PL).

Post Larva

Stockable PL in excellent quality will be available after 20-24 days. The crop of post larvae in the breeding tank is influenced by a number of factors like food availability, temperature solinity, pH etc. Phytoplankton is the food of post larvae.

Stocking PL into the ponds during the early morning or evening and keep the stocking density below 25/m^2.

Selection of FRY

Uniformity in size in a good indication that the fry must have come from the some batch and should be good quality. Size variation indicates the fry may have come from different batches or may have abnormal growth. Getting fry of different batches even of they are nearly equal in size should be avoided. Healthy fry will swim counter to current when the water in a basin is stirred. As the corrent subtides, the fry will cling to the side of the basin. It is not good sign it many of the fry are drown to words the centre.

Feeds

Table -2

Feeding rate of shnimps at different body wt (ABW) and type of feed :

ABW (gm)	Type of Feed	Feed rates. (% Biomars)
1 - 2	Starter	10 - 12
4	Starter	6.5
6	Grower	5.5
8	Grower	5.1
10	Grower	4.8
12	Grower	4.4
15	Grower	3.9
20	Finisher	3.5
25	Finisher	3.1
30	Finisher	2.7
35	Finisher	2.4.

Monitoring Feed Consumption

The ideal number of feeding trays per pond size is 4 for 0.5 ha and 6 for 1 ha. These feeding trays are basically utilized to monitor feed Constumption, and to assess feeding behaviour. shrimp condition and feed adjsutment. The amount of feeds consumed by the strimp will dictate whether to increase or decrease the quantity for the next feeding.

The following are as should be avoided in positioning the feeding trays.

(a) areas which are shunned by shrimps deel to possible toxicort including ammonia and state gorse.

(b) areas too close to pond edges where the pond bottom is uneven.

Feed tray allocation will be 0.5.1% from D.O.C. (days old culture) 1 to hamesh. Technician have the flexibility so adjust feed tray allocation within this range. Feeding time may be at 2AM, 6AM, 10AM, 2PM, 6PM, and 10PM, If feeding light times is necessary observe a feeding interval of 3 hours. Feed distribution must be 60% during PM feeding and 40% in AM. feeding.

Adjusting Feed Ratios

Weak of culture / Amount of feeds / day / 50, 000 try.

1. 1.5 kg for 7dyas

2. 2.3 kg for 7days

3. 2.3 kg + 150 gm in crement every day for 7days.

4. + 200gm increment every day for 7days of until 30th day of culture.

The following is the feeding guide for 2 gm and above.

Ideal feed = Total stock × SR% × ABW × Feeding Rate.

(SR - Stocking rate).

Feeding Management

Always maintain a stable healthy environment in the pond by keeping water quality parameters at their optimum level. Shrimps is good Condition Convert feed better and gain weight fasts. These a lower feed convertion rate (F.CR) can be obtained.

During molting period shrimps eat less than normal. Adjust feeding based on behaviour, Condition and demand of shrimp.

Table 3 : Water Parameters in the pond

Parameters	:	Ideal good condition at 0500Hrs. 11500Hrs.
Dissolved oxygen	:	4PPM. and above.
pH	:	7- 8.5.
3 Solinity	:	15PPL - 25 PPL.
Temperature	:	28 - 32^{0}C
Transparency	:	must be kept between 35 - 45 Cm.
Water depth	:	Must be maintained at 1.3m. average dept.
Water Colour	:	greenish brown to golden brown.
Ammonia	:	must be <10PPb> 100 PPb is dangerous.
Carbon dioxide	:	Normal <10PPM
1 nitrate	:	must be maitained <10PPb.
Hydrogen Sulphide	:	Below 0.00 7PPM. when pH drops <7.75 h_2S becomes dangerous.
Algal count	:	Maintain 75m and 100m cells / C.C.
Algalspevies	:	At least 5 Algal specil.

Changs of feed brand

New brand of Feed should changes slowly by 5 days, adding initially by mixing 1:1 and then grandually increase new brand if it is suitable.

Water exchanges

When the water detoriate, then it may be change by fresh one or may added Quantitative amount chemicals so standardise the quality of water.

Type of shrimp calture

Table (4) : Type of Prawn culture and Production

Item	Extensive	Modified Semi-Intensive	Semi-Intensiv	Intensive
PLAGE	PL 20	PL 20	PL 20	PL20
Stock Density				
Per m²	3-5	5-10	10-25	>25
Survival Rate %	<50	50-70	70-80	70-80
Water Exchange%	Minimal	10-15	25-30	>30
Feeds	Natural	Artificial	Artificial	Artificial
Aeration	Natural	Aerator	Aerator	Aerator
ABW (gm)	>35	33-35	33-35	30-33
DOC	90-120	120-150	120-150	120-150
Pond Prep days	-	30-45	30-45	30-45
Cycles	1.2	2	2	2
F.C.R	-	1.5-2.0	1.5-2.0	1.5-2.0
Yield/crop kg	150-500	500-1000	1000-5000	>5000
Production				
Cost / kg Rs.	30-50	50-100	100-200	>120

Pond Water Parameters and growth

During culture, growth is a Continuous Process interrupted only during molting. Growth is the totality of several biochemical process occaring in the organisation which results in size and weight increase.

Diseases in shrimp

Common diseases found in the pond reared shrimps are viral diseases such as Monodon baculovirus (MBV) and infection Hemato poietic and Hypodermal Necrosis Virus (IHHNV). Bacterial diseases are coused by vibriosis filamentous bacteria and luminous becteria. Protozoann such as vote celln Ephelota, Zootamniun etc overgrowth in gills loads to hypoxia. Aflatoxicosis or red disease is covred by fungal growth from Aspergillus flaves.

Disease Control

Prevention of diseases can be effectively done by not giving stress to shrimp, maintaining the required water quality, selection good fly and stocking the density of stry. Use of antibiotics may be restricted to hatchery to prevent development of pathogenes.

Figure "A" is a typically growth curve of Penaeus monoden. The best growth rate abtained for p. monadon in efficiently run ponds. ranges from 1.3-0 4 gm per day.

Figure - A

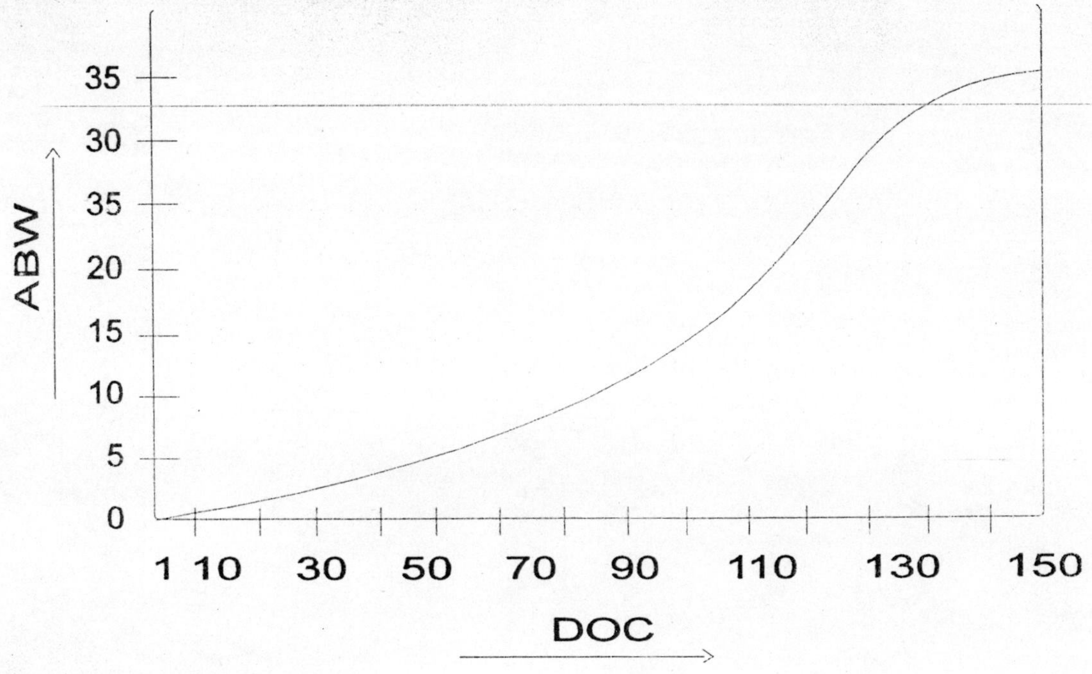

DOC. (Days old Culture)

ABW. (Average Body weight)

FCR. (Feed Conversion Rate).

Quality system for fish and fishery products

The future of the international fish trade is colsely tied up with the industry ability to comply with the extensive variety of food safety demands imposed by importing countries and satisfy the certification requirements of food control agencies in importing Countries.

Traditional method of inspection testing and training, serves only as monitoring devices. In order to promote international Trade and protech consumer's health and safety regulation are applied to seafoodin almost all Countries though a systematic cost effective and viable preventive quality system.

Prominent among the system concerning safety and health applicable to food products is Hauzard Analysis critical control points (HACCP) adopted by U.S.A., Canada and few other Countries EEC through specifically does not refsto H.A.C.CP but the principle refered to Article vi of the EEC Directive Number 91 / 493 / EEC States that management should identify critical points in their manufacturing process and should estabilist hand implements method for manufacturing and checking their critical points.

Under the joint FAO / WHO Codex standards programme codes for practices and product standard for food industry have been developed with the ultimate aim of providing guideline to the food industry in achieving a harmonization of the system.

Quality standard model I.S.O.9000

Pollution Control

It is require to put a Bio-pond for treatment of effluent water. Water should be treated by Bleaching powder to remove dark Colour and Coagulate the floating Insoluble material and make neutral water pH. Then aerate the water to make disired dissolve oxygen Concentration.

Preservation Technique

Prawn preserve by vaccum freeze drying technique or ordinary drying technique. There is a very good merit in vaccum freeze drying over ordinary drying. Though ordinary drying is cheaper processes rather than feeze drying process.

In vaccum freeze drying process one ton of prown produce 100 kg of freeze dried prawn and it produce again initial weight of prawn on rehydration.

But in case of Conventional drying method the product is obtained by dehydration and then rehydrated will produce only 200kg of prawn per ton of product.

Market

There is very good and prosperous market of quality products of aqua culture (Including prawn, sweet water fish, and Seafoods).

Table - I

Growth of marine fish production and seafood export

Year	Total Marine Fish Production in Tons (A)	Total Seafood in Tons (B)	% share of B to A.
1985	1534726	83651	5.45
1986	1707912	85843	5.02
1987	1647484	87179	5.89
1988	1775010	99777	5.62
1989	2221357	110243	4.96
1990	2189969	139419	6.36.

Table - II

Share of shrimp production in total Marine fish Product

Year	Total Marine Production in tons (A)	Total Shrimp Prooduction in tons (B)	% Share B to A
1985	1534726	121958	7.94
1990	2189969	122646	5.60.

Table - 3

Share of shrimp export in total seafood export

Year	Total seafood export in tons A	Total shrimp export in tons B	% Share of B to A
1985	83651	49681	50.39
1990	139419	63373	45.45

Table - 4

Trend Projection for Marine fish Production and seafood export by 2000 AD.

Year	Total Marine Fish Production (in tons)	Total see Food Productions quantity (in tons)	Export Value in crores
1991	2010419	172000	1375.00
1992	2072921	146219	1291.10
1993	2137365	155162	1494.72
1994	2203813	164653	1730.46
1995	2272327	174724	2003.38
1996	2342971	185411	2319.34
1997	2415811	196752	2685.73
1998	2490915	208786	3108.62
1999	2568355	221557	3598.89
2000	2648202	235108	4166.48.

Table - 5

Seafood Export Trend by 2000AD as a function of projected marine fish Production

Year	Total Marine Fish Production (Tons)	Total Seafood Exports. (Tons)
1994	2203813	140784
1995	2272327	147844
1996	2342971	155259
1997	2415811	163046
1998	2490915	171223
1999	2568355	179810
2000	2648202	188828

* *Above Tables are extracted from* ***Journal of Sea foods - Jan 94.***
By ***Dr. A. Yogumoorthi.*** *and* ***A. Sivashankar.***

Uses

It is rich source of animal protein. It is used for mal-nutrition. Fish protein concentrate has an important place amongst the protein cencentrates which may be used in large scale protein fortification on foods. It is the only animal protein concentrate, the production cost of which will compare with protein concentrates from vegetable sources, and it has a more balanced amino acid Composition. Only partially expleted fishery resources of the world, promise a continued supply of cheap raw material.

Table

Amino Acid Composition of Raw Material and Composite Fish Protein Concentrate Test sample

Amino Acid	Concertration	
	Raw sample	MPC Test sample
	percent of Protein (N X 6.25)	Percent of Protein (NX 6.25)
Lysine	7.40	8.41
Histidine	1.70	2.08
Arginine	6.08	7.13
Aspartic Acid	9.51	10.35
Threonine	4.15	4.47
Serine	4.11	4.65
Glutamic Acid	14.28	15.39
Protine	4.86	5.01
Glycine	7.82	8.09
Alanine	6.31	6.81
Valine	4.30	5.26
Methionine	3.05	3.30
Isoleacine	4.25	4.56
Leucine	7.06	7.78
Tyrosine	1.78	3.35
Phenylalanine	3.88	4.24
Tryptophan	0.68	1.03
Cystine	0.84	0.77.

Raw Matrial Suppliers

1. Zarcarias Liames Perea

   Lisepesca

   C/o Aguilas, 2 Poligono Aproin

   28320 PINTO, Madrid.

   Tel. : 6922523

   Fax : 6916766

2. Jean claude Greloud

   B.P. 119 - F 85602

   Montaigu Cedex.

   Tel. : (33) 51430303

   Tlx : 711076

   Fax : 51941965

3. Fisheries Development International Inc.

   108 Pleasant Hill Road.

   Chester, New Jersey,

   U.S.A. - 07930

   Tel. : 9088794250

   Fax : 908 - 8794712

4. M/S Apollo Sea foods

   Pvt.Ltd.Goa.

Manufacturer

1. Cham Marine Products Ltd.

   Bokhira - Porbander, 3605175

   Gujrat, India.

   Tel. : 91 - 286 - 22578, 23520

   Fax : 91 - 286 - 21404.

2. New Toyo Sea Foods Co Ltd.

   Ishikawa Building,

   20 - 1, 2 Chome,

   Misoki - cho, Chiyoda - KW,

   Tokyo, Japan.

   Tlx. : J 25220 - New, Food

   Fax : (03) 3263 - 6947

   Tel. : (03) 3262 - 4408.

3. Ameena Enterprises.

   Chandinoor - 688547

   Alappuzta - Distt,

   India.

   Tel. : 91- 47887 - 2630

   91 - 47887 - 2640

   Fax : 91 - 478872690

Address of Hetchery and Shrimp into product

1. N.C.C. Blue water Products Ltd.

   41, Nagarjuna Teids,

   Hyderabad - 500482

   Andhra Pradesh,

   India.

   Tel. : 33306, 228551, 227583,

   Tlx : 0425 - 2476,

   Fax : 040 - 226214.

2. Nekkant Sea foods Ltd,

   No - 62 Kirlampude Layont,

   Visakhapatnam - 530023.

   India.

   Tel. : (891) 54278, 55426,

   Tlx : (495) 433 Seta in,

   Fax : (891) 5559)

3. Falcon Marine exports Ltd.

   A/22 Cuttack Road,

   Ist Floor, Falcon House,

   Bhubaneswar -751006

   Orissa, India.

   Tel. : 50208, 54143,

   Tlx : 0678 - 6388 PRPIW.

   Fax : 0674 - 54105

Suppliers of Plant and Machinery

Pumps and valves

1. Yuken India Ltd.

   41 - 43 Lavelle Road,

   Bangalore - 560001

   Tel. : 213042.

2. Alweyn Pumps and System

   Pvt. Ltd.

   P.O. Box - 17421

   Bombay - 400059.

   Tel. : 6327467.

3. Watreat Engineers

   1/21, Rocky Industrial Estate.

   I.B. Patel Road,

   Goregoan (East)

   Bombay - 400063,

   Tel. : 685693,

   Tlx : 11 - 71099 - Hougein.

4. Acmevac Sales Pvt. Ltd

   109 Unique Industrial Estate

   Chakola Road,

   Andheri (East)

   Bombay - 400093

   Tel. : 6329647, 6300619.

   Tlx : 011-6425 ACME.

Ref *: India Sea food Trade Fair, Bombay, 10 - 13 Feb. 94*

Approximate Project Profile

Prawn Production in 5 Hectare Area.

1. (a) Land Required - 8 Hectare	:	Rs.800,000
(b) Land Development and Preparation of pond	:	Rs.1,600,000
2. Pump sets	:	Rs.200,000
3. Electricity Requirement	:	40 kwh.
4. Working Capital Required per annum	:	Rs.1,900,000
5. Production Cost / annum	:	Rs.2,581,250
6. Sales Turnover / annum (Rs 125/kg)	:	Rs.3,125,000
7. Profit per annum	:	Rs.543750
8. Fixed Cost	:	Rs.1,000,000
9. BEP%.	:	35.22

Assumption

(1) Prawn Production will be 5 tonnes / hectare.

(2) Sales Price Rs. 125 /kg.

References

1. Dr. A. Jogomoorthi and A. Shivashankar - Sea food Journnal - Jan 94 page - 27- 33

2. T.K. Chatterjee - Marine Aqua and

Research centre.

Zoological Survey of India,

Digha - 721428 - W.B.

Journal of Sea food Export

Feb - 1995 Volu XXVI No 2

Page - 23 - 27

3. Pro A.N. Bose - Fish Protein Concentrate

Protein Fortification of foods

Association of Food technologists Eastern Regional Branch.

Reference :

Aquaculture

1. Complete Library of the garden

   The Readers digest

   Volume I - Volume 3.

2. Survey of Rose growing centres

   and Rose industry in India -

   C.S.I.R. - V. Narayan Swamy

   And K. Biswas - 1957.

3. An encyclopedia of annual and

   Biennial Garden Plants - charles - 0 - Booth.

6 FLORICULTURE

Introduction

Flowers in room have a quality in common with the presence of the people or of a fire. They bring the room to life, make it look lived in. The eye leaps to a vase of flowers, leaps to something living and colourful ...... and if, on nearer view, you find beauty of line, detail colour blending and satisfying balance, your pleasure is so much the greater.

The outline of any flower group is influenced by the shape of the vase and find the simplest way to get the outline clear is to place in position two or three flowers to indicate the general shape, putting in first the highest central flower and then the two sides or for carnulopia or sauce boot, putting the highest and the lowest of flowers, or for a centre piece on a table to fix the total length,then within the framework, to build up the whole.

World flower industry is registering a fast rate of growth. In 1991 it was estimated that more than US $100 billion worth of cut flowers internationally traded.International trade is in respect of more than 30,000 varities of orchids, thousands of varities of roses, carnation, chrysanthemum, lilies and begonias.

Because of the developments in biotechnology, the demand pattern for flowers and ornamental plants is also changing. The consumers are looking for something new, may be yellow and blue anthurium, black and blue roses, fragnant gladiolus and so on.

Commercial floriculture is the most profitable agro-industry in many developed and developing countries. For example, Dutch economy is dependent upon Tulip and other flower crops. Developing countries like Israel, Thailand, Colombia, Malaysia, Singapore, Sri Lanka, Keneya and Mexico are earning a sizable part of their foreign exchange from the flower industry.

India has many opportunities for the development of commercial floriculture industry, thanks to the progress made by biotechnology industry in the country. It is estimated that India's share in the global flower and ornamental plants is much less than 1%.

Rapid strides have been made in the field of micro propogation of ornamental plants. This has been made possible largely by private laboratries and commercial nurseries. Among the ornamental plants which have been micropropogated are Anthurium, Begonia, Cattleya, Dendrobium, Daisy, Dahlia, Gerbera, Chrysanthemum, Gladiolus and many others.

From the international trade point of view, the following flowers and ornamental plants are significant. Rose, Carnation, Chrysanthemum, Orchid, Gladiolus, Snapdragon and Tulip among the major cut flowers. All the minor cut flowers, Gerbera, Anthurium, Gypsophila, Iris, Nareissus, Statice or Sea Lavender are made. There is also demand for potted flowering plants. These include Chrysanthemum, African Violets, Begonia, Geranium and Kalanchoe.

The Water Garden

A group of nymphaeas(water lilies) are the best known of aquatic. They grow to various size and are suitable for all types of pool.

These types of flowers planted in the pool. Pool may be rectangular or square base. It should be observed that water of the pool should not be polluted by any old leaves or dirty material. It should be in the open land where full sun shine will be fallen.

There are three ways of dealing with the problem

1. By keeping the pool full of the water for six months, then emptying and rinsing it out before planting. This is the usual procedure with pool constructed in the autumn.

2. By pointing over the surface with one of the several proprietary insulating substance available from sundriesmen. Most of these substances also contain a water tightness.

3. By neutralizing with acid and alkaline substances which come from the cement. Any cheap acid such as commercial syrupy, phosphoric acid does for this purpose. Stir into the water enough to show and acid reaction to litmus paper 24 hrs after adding. Constantly moving water is not good for lilies.

Many plants like to feel influence of water without actual growing in it, they can not stand drought, yet can not live in stagnant moisture.

Bag plants in reasonably moist or heavy soils sufficient moisture is usually present in the ground to take care of their needs. An annual top dressing with a mutch of well rotted leaves will conserve the moisture.

Planting

Water lilies need very good rich composition manure for getting good results.

Time of Planting

From March to end of the May or 1st week of June.

Trouble In The Water

Aphids or greenfly are the chief pest to attack water plants. The attacks may be saved by using BHC or nicotine solution over the flower when there is no fish in the pool.

Another method of destroying aphids is to lay hoops or similar shaped pieces of metal over the crowns of the water lilies so that the leaves and flowers are forced beneath the water. Leave them overnight and by morning all the aphids will be drawned or consumed by fish.

One year covred cow dung is best manure for water lilies.IT should be careful that compost manure formed by cow dung should not contain excess minerals which helps grow Algae more. Do not use excess organic manure which decomposes and produce bubbling in the pool to cause of suffocation towards fish.

In absence of compost manure of cow dung we can use coarse bone meal.

Discoloured Water

Green or cloudy water is the chief worry of the cultivator and is caused either by stirred up mud or sediment ,or by misoscopic plant.

Cleaning

From time to time small pools need to be empted and replanted, chiefly because the lilies will have exhausted the soil and flowers will have become fewer and smaller.

Planting Of Rhododendron

Rhododendrons will grow only on an acid soil. If lime or chalk is present in any form there is little hope of success, except by making up banks of special soil or by growing them in pots or tubs. There are many ways in which to discover if soil is suitable for Rhododendrons. (1) One is by soil testing (2) By observing the growth of vegetation.If there is growth of gorse, heather, pine trees and silver birch is indicating of soil acidity.

Planting

Rhododendron prepare a hole deep enough to bring the old planting mark on the stem level with the soil surface.Put peat or leaf mould round the roots, fill in the hole and tread down firmly.

Or dig the ground well and work in some well rotted cow manure or lime free compost.This should be done a month before planting which may be at any time in open weather from the end of september to the middle of april.

Pick the dead flowers as soon as they are over.This will allow the new growth to develop and form next year's flower buds.In the spring give a mulch of peat or leaf mould, mixed with well rotted cow manure, if available.

The Rhododendron is the most decorative of all evergreen flowing shrubs.Rhododendron was called Alpine Rose in Great Britain. Flowers of Rhododendrons are available from January to August in all colours from pure white to a dark purple that is almost black.

Rose

For good cultivation of rose, soil should contents this following constituents:

pH	6.4 - 81.
soluble solts	0.5 - 1.72
Organic Nitrogen	0.042 - 0.112%
K_2O	0.27 - 0.89%
P_2O_5	0.12 - 0.40%
COO	0.5 - 2.0%
MgO	0.2 - 12.0%
Fe_2O_3	0.7 - 4.0%
Al_2O_3	1.3 - 3.5%
SiO_2	0.087 - 0.2%

Rose tree should planted under full sun shine.Plantation time is March, October and December.Flowering starts about eight months after planting land should be moistened by water and temperature variation may be good for cultivation of Rose 20°C - 35°C.

Usually 5000 - 10,000 plants per area can be planted in a well prepared land

Land Preparation

Cut out the land centrally to make trench 3'depth and 2'width.Heap the clay in one side, fill up the trench by old leaves to one feet then by manure of NH_4SO_4 or nitratate or phosphate by 1' then by available soil.Prepare this land for 8 month - 12 months before Rose plantation.

Recommended fertilise per Rose trees 2gms after 15 days interval.

Pest And Disease

Especially fungal diseases are attacked in the Rose plant.It can be removed by cutting the portion of the plant which is attacked by the diseases and then sprayed by dilute sovlon solution or by dilute lysoes solution or by sulphate of iron at the rate of an ounce per gallons of water.

The production of rose starts from March to December.

Bellis

They are low growing herbs. They require a moist, rich soil and flower with great freedom from May to July. The flowers are charming for cutting and last a long time in water. They make attractive plants for winter flowering in the cool green house.

For bedding out, seed should be sown in a reserve border in June and covered to a depth of one quarter of an inch. Germination takes place in about ten days and the young plants should be pricked out 3inches apart. Plant out in September or the following April, allowing 6inches between each plant. Alternatively, sow the seed in September when they are to flower and thin out to required distance apart.

They may also be grown as annuals and for these purpose seed should be sown under glass in March and germinated in a temperature of 55 - 60°F. When large enough to handle, the young plants should be pricked out 2 inches apart in boxes and grown on at a slightly lower temperature. Harden off in April and plant out in May spacing them 4 inches apart.

For winter flowering under glass, seed should be sown in June or July and the young plants pricked off into 3 inches pots. Grow on in cold frame during the summer, and when necessary, pot up finally into 4 inches pots. Transfer to a cool green house in October and grow on at a temperature of 50 - 55°F watering sparingly and vertilating the green house whenever possible.

B.Rotundifolia (Syn Belliumrotundifolium)

A most attractive species from North Africa, with long stalked, deeply toothed, oval or slightly heart shaped leaves and snowy white flowers, each measuring about one and quarter inches in diametre.

Diseases

Grey Mould Attack

Light brown spots or blotches, covered with a dense grey mould appear on the leaves, stens and flowers.The plants frequently wilt and if all attacked at the base may collapse.

Control

Burn infected plants and spray the remainder with Bordeaux mixture to prevent spread.Avoid high humidities under glass.Flowering plants may be sprayed with disodium ethylene, bis dithio carbonate since this causes less damage to the petals than Bordeaux mixture, and a tetrachloronitrobenzeen dust has also proved very effective.More recently griscofulvin an antibiotic, has been used systematically to afford healthy plants resistance to attack.

ANDROSACE : ROCK JASMINE PRIMULACEAL

These are small herbs with tafted basal, entire or toothed leaves and short scapes of purple, pines, red or white, solutary or umbellate flowers. The flowers resemble those of Primula but differ in the corolla being shorter than the calyx and constricted at the throat. None of species are sun lavers and appreciate a position on a northerly scope or in partical shade.

Before plantin out it is advisable to incorporate peat, leafmould or well-rolted manure with the soil to ensure a high moisture content during the summer. without moist conditions at the roots they must be done corefully, however, since they are equally resentful of water logged conditions but on well-drained gritty soils rich in humus they express their approval of such treatment with a profusion of small but very attaractive flowers.

A few of the species make charming plants for spring and summer flowering in the cold green house, and for this purpose they should be grown in shallow pans, covered on the surface with small pieces of broken rock.

Seed should be shown on the surface of the compost and the container watered by immersion cover with a sheet of glass and germinate in a temparature of 50 - 55°F. Germination is sometimes slow and irregular and it is always adviseble to use fresh seed. As soon as the young plants are large enough to handle, they should be pricked out two inches apart in boxes and grown on in of first proof green house or frame.

These are different varieties of species which can grown in the open garden in different season.

Process Flow Diagram

Selection of land

↓

Preparation of land

↓

Harvesting of lands

↓

Observation of plant growth

↓

Spraying of pesticides

↓

Changing the water if required

↓

Bud or flower Appearance

↓

Collection of bud or flower or leaves

↓

Pack in polypack

↓

Store in refrigeration

↓

Marketing by transporting

↓

Through refrigerated van.

Plant and Machinery Suppliers

(A) Plant Growth Chambers :

1. Heraeus Instrument GmbH

   411 International Trade Tower

   Nehru Place,

   New Delhi - 110019

   India.

   Tel. : 091-11-6424038,
   6469568.

   Fax : 091-11-6466721.

2. Precision Analytical Instruments. Pvt. Ltd.

   3 - B, Pusa Road,

   New Delhi - 110005,

   India.

   Tel. : 091-11-5738169.

   Fax : 091-11-5754489

(B) Pumps

3. ASR Instruments

   Baba Chambers,

   73 Richmond Road,

   Bangalore - 560025,

   India.

   Tel. : 091-80-2212748

   Fax : 091-80-5583539.

4. HETO HOLTEN DENMARK

   Gydewang 17 - 19,

   DK - 3450 Allerod,

   DENMARK.

   Tel. : 4548142777

   Fax : 40037.

(C) Refrigeration equipment

5. Blue Star Ltd.

   Sahas 414 / 2,

   Veer Savarkar Marg,

   Prabhadevi,

   Bombay - 400025.

   India.

   Tel. : 091-22-4306155.

   Fax : 011-71193.

6. Labindia Instruments Pvt. Ltd.

   M - 2 Pal Mohan Sadan.

   26 / 32 Patel Nagar,

   New Delhi - 110008.

   India.

   Tel. : 091 - 11 - 5723822

   Fax : 091 - 11 - 5751066.

Suppliers of Raw Material

1. M/s Unicorn Biotek Ltd,

   1-10-44/1/1 Chikoti Gardens,

   Begunpet,

   Hyderabad - 500016

2. M/s Cadila Laboratories Ltd,

   Ghodasar,

   244 Mani Nager

   Post Box No. - 9004,

   Ahmedabad - 380008

3. M/s Indrayani Biotech Ltd.

   Pune.

Uses

The uses of flower as traditional offerings to gods and goddeses for decorative purposes particularly on festival occasions and also for personnel adomments has been prevailing in India since long.

Flowers have also been used as a raw material for perfumary products and various medicinal preparations.

The use of cut flowers with long stems and potted plants for decorative purposes.

Plant Machineries requirement for floriculture

(1) Pumps.

(2) Deep tubewells orwater reservoir.

(3) Defferent Type of seissors or cutting instrument.

(4) Spraying Machine.

(5) Hand Tract or Tractor.

(6) Chessels.

(7) Lighting System

(8) Cooling Tower or Refrigeration System.

Test Parameters

It should always be tested that seed used for floriculture product be well developed hybridised seed or from developed plant tissueculture such that product which will comes out can compete with international market requirement. Growth of the plant will be rapid and output from the product will be economic viable for international market competition in required quality.

Pollution Control

In case of fluoriculture production these is no pollution produced. Perhaps floriculture procedure will save the enfiroment by purifying polluted air to nonpolluted air.

Preservation Technique

Flowers and decorative leaves are very delicious item. These have very small self life. Some of the flowers in dry form has longer self life. Self life of flower can be increased by stoning of law tempies below 4°C. Flowers and leaves can be stared in refrigeration room. Transportation of flowers and leaves should be done by refrigerated van.

Market studies on floriculture

The study Covers non flowering (green) foliage plants fresh decorative cut foliage classified under the following headings in the Brussels Tariff Nomenculture (BTN) and the standard international trade Classification (SITC)

SITC	BTN	Description
291.69	06.02	Other live plants (including trees, shrubs, branches, roots, cuttings and slipes.
292.71	06.03	Cut flowers and flower buds fresh dried, dyed, bleached, impregnated or otherwise prepared.
292.72	06.04	Foliage branches and other parts (other than flowers or buds) of trees, shrubs, bushes and other plants and mosses, lichens and grasses being goods of a kind suitable for bouquets or ornamental purposes fresh, dried dyed bleached, impregnated or otherwise prepared.

The study reviews products that one of special interest to developing countries wishing to develop and export-oriented floricultural industry. That of the items under the SITC / BTN categories listed above, it limits it's coverage to green plants (as opposed to lichens and mosses) in such forms as cuttings, canes, and large indoor plants It exclude flowering plants, shrubs and bushes. Although dried flowers may be of interest to several developing countries, the study focuses exclusively on fresh cut flowers simlarly, it deals only with fresh cut foliage.

Objective and limitation

(1) *To diversify the exports of floriculture products.*

Supply and Demand

The federal republic of Germany is the world's largest importer of all categories of *floricultural products.*

Federal Republic of Germany

Imports and export of cut flowers, decorative cut foliage and pot plants 1991 - 1995.

Year / Product	Imports	Exports
cut flowers		
1991	2006.2	46.42
1992	2206.82	48.5
1993	2648.18	50.0
1994	3310.23	49.5
1995	3000.0	52

Decorative cut foliage

1991	108.78	5.18
1992	119.65	5.439
1993	120.25	5.98
1994	132.28	6.34
1995	145.51	6.59

Pot Plantes

1981	247.3	23.7
1982	286.6	25.2
1983	319.9	28.1
1984	335.0	30.6
1985	384.7	34.8.

Cut Flowers

Category	1981	1985
Carnation	955.5	848.6
Roses	537.6	708.0
Chrysan muners	266.5	281.9
Gladali	89.9	72.7
Other	6247.0	66,295.0.

(a) Excluding reindeer moss christmas trees and conifor branches.

(b) Excluding flowering plants with buds or flowers.

Demand decline considerably in the month of May-September.

Customer preference is larger flowered with long stem, Red coloured.

INVESTMENT : ROSE

Project Size : Three Hectares

	Rs. In Lakhs		Rs. per sq. m.	
Description	1	2	1	2
Greenhouses	75.0	135.0	250	450.0
Cooling System	-	60.0	-	200.0
Watering Installation	30.0	30.0	100.0	100.0
Buildings	75.0	75.0	250.0	250.0
Truck	15.0	15.0	-	-
Miscallaneous	39.0	63.0	130.0	210.0
Total	234.0	378.0	730.01	210.0

1. Pune, Nasik, Bangalore

2. Hyderabad, New Delhi, Punjab

INVESTMENT : CARNATION

Project Size : Three hectares

	Rs. in Lakhs		Rs. Per sq. m.	
Description	1	2	1	2
Greenhouses	60.0	120.0	200.0	400.0
Cooling System	-	60.0	-	200.0
Watering Installation	22.5	22.5	75.0	75.0
Buildings	45.0	45.0	150.0	150.0
Truck	15.0	15.0	-	-
Miscellaneous	28.5	52.5	95.0	175.0
Total	171.0	315.0	520.0	1000.0

1. Pune, Nasik, Bangakore

2. Hydrabad, New Delhi, Punjab

Project Profile

Floriculture

Product Rose Flower (used as planted Trees - 10, 000, cut flower)

1.	Land used :	10, 000 sq Meters.
2.	Cost of Land + Cost Built up area + land Development cost :	Rs. 57, 50, 000
3.	Plant Machinery cost :	Rs. 1, 00, 00000
4.	Other Fixed Expenditure :	Rs. 5, 00000
5.	Total Fixed Capital Required :	Rs. 1, 62, 50000
6.	Raw Material per annum :	Rs. 55, 00, 000/-
7.	Labour per Annum :	Rs. 8, 00, 000/-
8.	Other office expenditure :	Rs. 6, 00, 000/-
9.	Working Capital Require/annum :	Rs. 69, 000; 00/-
10.	T.C.I. :	Rs. 17975000/-
11.	Production Cost :	Rs. 10196250/-
12.	Sales Turnover :	Rs. 1, 31, 40, 000
13.	Profit / annum :	Rs. 2943750/-
14.	Fixed Cost :	Rs. 60, 36, 250/-
15.	BEP % :	67.21.
16.	Profit % with T.C.I. :	16.37%

7 TISSUE CULTURE

Introduction

This is one of the best in the field of agriculture. Though Tissue culture plants found out in 1940's but it's wide application starts only few years back, Now it is realize all over world, tissue culture is the process to preserve the every good necessary plants through laboratory scale to field origine. Tissue culture is the process to develop the plants very rapidly in artificial way with a very good uniform manner.

Tissue culture involves production of genetically identical plant progeny through the cloning on a vegetative Tissue or organ of the parent plant or ex-plants on nutrient medium containing growth harmones under sterile condition.The cultures are kept under controlled conditions of light and temperature suiting the particular plant species to yield plant lets. This plantlets after hardening in green house can be transfred to the fields.

There requirements of sterile media for the development of plantlets from plant's tissues. Sterile media means it is completly free from microbes and viruses. Every media contains water, it should be careful to make water microbes free, mineral free, and pryrogen free.

Metrient media for plant tissue culture means the media contains all the minerals, elements, vitamins and growth factors which are required for the formation of tissues to plantlets and plantlets to plant.

After chromosorne replication, a cell divides to produce daughter cell. This method of increasing cell number is a uniparental (asexual) process called vegetative reproduction. starting with single. organism, contineous vegetative reproduction results in a population of cells called a clone, barning mutations, all members of a clone are geneficly identical. If mutation occurs during clonal growth the nutant in transmitted to all the progeny of the mutant cell, thus producing a genetically mosaic clone whose proportion of mutant individuals varies, depending upon the fine the mutation occurred and the relative reproductive potential of mutant and nonmutant cells.

Tissue culture is the process of rapid vegetative multiplication of super clones.

Cultivation Process

Selection of high producing cell lines for a plant tissue culture is dependent on two fectors, that the starting meterial is heterogeneous strain and that a high percentage of the cells are stable for a long period of time.

Once plant cells (strain) has been identified it should stored in nutrient media aseptically in presence of liquird nitrogen will be used as master lot. From the master lot one lot will be used as working lot. Very aseptically fromworking lot transfer the cells (Biomolecules) in a test tube contains sterile nutrient media keep it for about 7 days at temperature 30°C with sterile air circulation. In the test tube there will be cells growth, after proper growth appears, it is again transfer to erlenmeyer flask containing sterile nutrint media again keep it for few days (may be about 7 days)again these will be increaseof cells con-centration. Now this cells may transfer to cell culture vesself afeptically to for the growth cell culture vessel. Contains liquid nutrient media, air lift system agitation system, pH control system, temperature control system. In the cell culture vessel cells will be grown up from 4 gm. fresh at to 300gm fresh wt.

This cells are seperated very aseptically such that each cell will be microbial contamination free and should be damaged free. (Nutrient media content corbon source may be glucose, nitrogen source urea, ammonium sulphate or ammonium nitrate, vitamins, growth factors trace minerals like zinc, cobalt, cupper and iron)

This cells (super clones) used for rapid vegetative growth.

This sterilised cells or mother surface sterile mother plant is put in test tube containing sterile solid nutrient agar media (15-20 ml in 40 ml. tubes) with cotton plug. Each tube put in a test tube rack and keep the tubes in sterile room of 30°C, with 60 -80 % Humidity and sterile air flow rate

10 -20 L.P.M, wait for few days (3-7days or more) the cells or mother plants multiplied and growth appears in a test tube.

When growth will appears, this growth again fraster aseptically to jar containing solid sterile agar media, keep the Jars on the rack of a room maintaining temperature 28 - 30°C, strile air flow rate 20 - 25 L.P.M. and humidity maintain 70 - 75% and also controlled light reflection (Jar volume will be 500 ml and nutrient media content 50 ml.)

When adequate shoots and roots are develop in the plant lets it is then transfer to polytunnels containg preplanned sterile fertile media. Keep this tunnel in the artificial room where proper lighting air flow rate (30 40 L.P.M), Humidity maintain 70 - 80% temperature maintained 30°C and also shedding arrangement in the room.

This plantlets will keep for one month in the poly funnels for further development.

These plantlets are distributed to the planters. Planters keep this plantlets in the nursery for six month before transplanting to the main field.

By that above way it is possible to produce 1000 or more unifom plants at a fine.

Process flow sheet

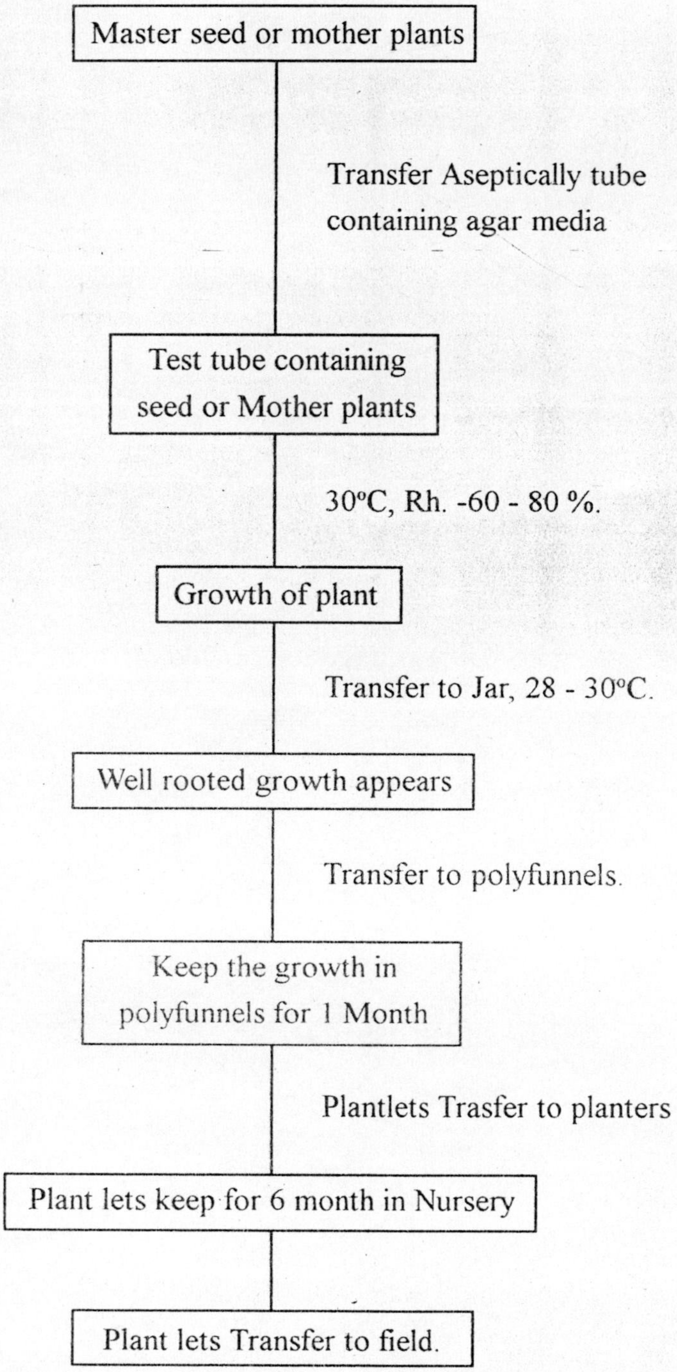

Plant and machinery Required

1. Laminar Air flow station.

2. Prefilter, Micro "V" filter, and Hepa filter.

3. Air handling unit.

4. Artificial Room for garden.

5. Cooling Tower.

6. Special Type of lighting and heating arrangament.

7. Fiber glass Trays, Polypropyfene trays.

8. Tissue culture flask, Ptridisk, erlenmeyer flask.

9. Culture vessel with special oxygen entry line.

10. Pumps, Compressons, special type grills.

11. Roc

Suppliers of plant and Machinery

Suppliers of Laminar work station

1. Klenzaids Bioclean Devices (P) Ltd.

A - 21, MIDC, Street No - 3,

Andheri (East)

Bombay - 400093

India.

2. John Fowler India Limited.

Sarjapur Road,

Bangalore - 560034.

India.

Tel. : 091 - 80 - 5530026,
5534539.

Tlx : 0845 - 2545.

Fax : 091 - 80 - 5533228.

3. Astec Environmental Systems Ltd.

31 Lynx Crescent

Weston - Super - Mare

BS24 9DJ

Tel. : 0934 - 418685

Tlx : 444181.

Prefilter, Micro-V - filter, HEPA Filter

4. Filtech pharmalab Pvt. Ltd.

   Star metal Compound.

   L.B.S. Marg

   Vikhroli (West)

   Bombay - 400083,

   India.

   Tel. : 091 - 22 - 5782559 / 5631

   Tlx : 011 - 71934.

   Fax : 022 - 5785329.

5. Labmate (Asia) Private Limited.

   Lokesh Towers,

   18, Kodambakkam High Road

   Madras - 600034.

   India.

   Tel. : 091 - 44 - 8283782

   Tlx : 041 - 7558.

   Fax : 09 - 44 - 8256971

Air Handling unit

6. S.K. System Private Ltd.

7. Blue Star Limited.

   Band Box House,

   Prabhadevi,

   Bombay - 400025.

   Tel. : 4933101

   Fax : 91 - 22 - 4933799.

   Tlx : 011 - 71071

Cooling Tower

8. PAHARPUR COOLING TOWERS (P) Ltd.

   8 /1 /B Diamond Harbour Road.

   Calcutta - 700027.

Fiber Glass Trays and Polypropylene Trayes and Tissue culture wares

9. TARSONS PRODUCTS

818 Marshall House,

33 /1. N.S. Road

Calcutta - 700001

Tel. : 220-4022, 220-9025,

21-1013.

Fax : 033 - 211014.

10. JAGKUMAR & COMPANY

BIOTECHNOLOGY DIVISION.

Purshattam Bhawan,

1/3 Issaji Street,

Vadgadi,

Bombay - 400003

Tel. : 346264, 323451,

Tlx : 011 - 76960 Topin.

11. CHEMTRON ANALYTICAL INSTRUMENTS LTD.

306, 9/2 East Patel Nagar,

New Delhi - 110008

India.

Tel. : 091 - 11 - 5755987

Fax : 091 - 11 - 5724135.

12. KPS Scintific Products Company.

D - 64, 65 Amar Colony,

Lajpat Nagar.

New Delhi - 110024

India.

Tel. : 091 - 11 - 6425156

Fax : 091 - 11 - 6425156

13. Flow Laboratories Ltd

P.O. BOX - 17

Decond Ave Industrial Estate,

IRVUNE AYRSHIRE

SCOTLAND KA 12 BNB

Tel. : (0294) 74242

Tlx : 77231 FLOW - G.

14. GENETIC RESEARCH INSTRUMENTATION LTD.

Gene House, Dunmow Road.

FELSTED,

Dunmow, Essex CM 63LD

Tel. : 0371 - 821082

Tlx : 937400 ONECOM G 32257001.

15. Gibco Limited.

P.O. BOX - 35

Trident House

Rentrew Road, PAISLEY,

Scotland, PA3 4EF.

Tel. : 041 - 889 - 6100.

Tlx : 777968 / 777029.

Suppliers of Raw Materials.

Tissue culture Media

1. Flow Laboratories Ltd.

   P.O. BOX - 17

   Second Ave Industrial Estate,

   IRUINE, AYRSHIRE.

   SCOT LAND, KA 12 8NB.

   Tel. : (0294) 74242.

   Tlx: 77231 FLOWG.

2. Sisco Research Laboratories Pvt. Ltd.

   2F /C Satam Industrial Estate

   Cardinal Gracious Road,

   Andheri (E)

   Bombay - 400009.

   India.

   Tel. : 091 - 22 - 8323882

   Fax : 091 - 22 - 8380998.

3. K.P.S. Scientific Products Company

   D-64, 65 Amar Colony

   Lajpat Nagar,

   New Delhi - 110024

   INDIA.

   Tel. : 091 - 11 - 6425156

   Fax : 091 - 11- 6425156.

Manufacturers

1. A.V. Thomos and Co Ltd

   P.B.NO - 1685,

   28 / 961 Panam Pilly Nagar,

   Cochin - 682015.

2. Indo - Americam Hybrid Seeds Biotech Division.

   P.B. NO - 7099

   Banashamkari II Stage

   Banglore - 604940, 606479,

   Tel. : 604940, 606479,

   Tlx : 0845 8204 IAHS IN.

3. Hindustan Lever Ltd.

   165 /166 backbay Reclamation

   Bombay - 400020

4. M/s Tata Tea Ltd.

   1. Bishop Zafroy Road,

   Calcutta - 700020.

5. Indo French Bio farm (P) Ltd.

   6 - 3 - 862 Ameerpet.

   Hyderabad - 500016.

Address of Technology Available

1. Biotech Consortium India Ltd.

   Kundan House, 4th floor,

   16, Nehru Place.

   New Delhi - 110019.

   Tel. : 6415385, 6415314.

   Telex : (031) - 71209 BCIL IN.

   Fax : (011) 6438926.

2. M / S Sunki Privete Ltd.

   Brisbane

   Australia

3. Sterlin Limite.

   Sterlin House

   Clock House lane

   FEL THAM

   Middx TW 14BQS.

   Tel. : 0794 -251155

   Tlx : 8812910.

Test Parameters

Plants are tested by field trials.

Market Study

There will be very good market demand of tissue culture Process product. Since in future there is requirement of rapid growth of plants and production of fruits and vegetables to keep space with the requirementof the vast growth of human being. It is also necessary to produce required crops and vegetables within limited land. Since land availability in limited according to increase the population.

Uses and Advantages

(1) It is uses for improving crops quality and uniformity.

(2) It helps to produces superior plants of different agro elimaticzine.

(3) The plants are generally resistant to pest and disease.

(4) The plants produces greater output.

(5) It helps to preserve all the plant's origin.

Approximate Cost Analysis

Tissue culture products

1. **Production**	:	2 million plant lets / annum
2. **Fixed Capital Required**	:	
(a) Land + Built up area	:	Rs.42,50,000
(b) Plant and Machinery	:	Rs.37,00,000
(c) Other Fixed Expenditure	:	Rs.10,50,000
		Rs.90,00,000
3. **Working Capital Required**	:	
(a) Raw Material / annum	:	Rs.1,80,00,000
(b) Salary wages / annum	:	Rs.18,00,000
(c) Miscllaneous Recurring area expenditure / annum	:	Rs.98,80,000
		Rs.2,96,80,000
4. **Total Capital Investment**	:	
(a) Fixed Capital	:	Rs. 96,00,000
(b) 3 Months Working Capital	:	Rs.74,20,000
		Rs.1,64,20,000

(5) **Project Cost** :

(a) Fixed Capital	:	Rs.90,00,000
(b) 1/4 of 3 Months W/C	:	Rs.18,55,000
		Rs.1,08,55,000
6. **Production Cost/annum**	:	Rs.3,28,10,499
7. **Turn over by sales of 2 million plant lets** (at the Rate Rs. 20 /each)	:	Rs.40,000,000
8. **Profit / annum**	:	Rs.71,89,501
9. **Fixed Cost / annum**	:	Rs.15,002,499
10. **B.E.P.%**	:	Rs.67.6
11. **Profit % on T.C.I.**	:	Rs.43.6%

References

(1) Plant cell suspension culture theology wagon R Curtis : Department of Chemical / Biotechnical Institute.

Pennsylvania , State university, University park, pennsylvania: 16802 Journal of Biotechnology and Bioengineering - volume 42, Page - 520 - 526, 1993.

(2) Plant culture vessel - comprises rockwood or cellulose fibermass carrier and filter for polyphenol removal befor culture medium recycle.

Tokimaka JP 5049 - 358 - 21.08.91, - JP

2092 63 (02. 03. 90). 21. 0891 or 209263. 91 - 111 781/19.

(3) J2 Plant cell drug from plant cell and Tissue culture - culture vessel design for pharmacutical production in plant cell culture and Tissue culutre.

Kreis W.Pharma, Zeutrerches Institute, Aufder Magensteas and 7400, Tuebiujen, Germany, DHCH Apothzir (1993) 133, 15. 17 - 18. 21 - 22 - 28 - 35 - 36, 394.

(4) Tissue culture Pilot Plant - Udyog Yug, FEBRUARY - 1995. Page 24 - 25.

8 BULK DRUGS AND DRUG INTERMEDIATE

INTRODUCTION

Drugs are basically special chemical Compound or live cells or dead cells or protein bodies or neucleic acid which have property to attack disease producing microbes to kill the microbes or stop the activity of microbes such that disease cannot be sprayed in lives. Drugs or Drugs intermediates are produced from basic raw materials may be chemical, plant origin or live cells.

It can be industrially manufacture by maintaining very careful process parameters. (That is Temperature, pH, Catalyst, time of Reac-tion, use of solvents, even also design parameters of reactors etc)

Most drugs are lost their activity at high temperature (i,e) greater than 50°C) even at 30°C also. It is necessary to preserve drugs at low temperature for long days storage. Drugs and drug intermediates are high molecular weight compound.

Now a days drugs produced by biotechnology base is much more interested and much more beneficial to the society world is search for some products which can stop or recover of heart attack or recover cancer diseases etc.

Vaccins are most important drugs produced by live cells which are much more important in modern development.

Ephidrin Hydrochloride

Manufacturing Process

Ephidrine hydrochloride manufactured by two stage of Synthetic Process. First pepared phenyl acetyl carbinol and then it is transformed to ephidrin hydrochloride.

Preparation of Phenyl Acetyl carbinol or ketol

Raw Material required of following composition (weight percent basis).

Molasses	-	12%
(Sugar content 44%)		
Baker's yeast	-	2.4%
Water	-	84.44%
NH_4 SO_4	-	0.06%
Vitamin B_1	-	—
Benzaldehyde	-	1 - 10%
Aeration rate	-	5 - 10 L.P.M.
Temp	-	30.32^{o}C.
pH of Media	-	5 - 5.6.

Procedure

Took molasses in fermentor and diluted to 12 % by sterile water and then added to the fermentor ammonium sulfate and vitamin B_1 required amount. Start aeration to the fermentor at the rate of 5 - 10 L.P.M. Total. Addition of Benzaldehyde to the fermentor be divided into 5 equal parts whithin 4 Hours. After last addition of Benzaldehyde, wait for one hour before starting extraction of the fermented broth. If required add 240 ml of acetaldehyde to the fermentor by last two stage of addition. Phenyl acetyl carbinol produced in the fermented broth will be around 1.4 - 1.5%. Leave phenyl acetyl carbinol is the active ketol which is used for conversion of ephidrine hydrochloride. Total time of conversion will take 7 - 10 Hours.

Extraction of Phenyl Acetyl Carbinol

Took fermented broth in the column reactor. Extraction of the broth done by using benzene as solvent. Took benzene in close vessel and start extraction by (flame proof pump) circulation of benzene through reactor to benzene recover to pump. Extraction Continued for forty minutes to extract out phenyl acetyl carbinol. Extraction carried out at 30 - 35°C.

Recovery of Phenyl acetyl carbinol :

Now took phenyl acetyl carbinol extract with benzeen in distillation column to seperate benzene (solvent) and phenyl acetyl carbinol. In distillation column temperature should not increase more than 50°C.

Preparation of Ephidrine hydrochloride

For the preparation of ephidrine following raw materials required .

Phenyl Acetyl chloride	:	25%
Benzeen	:	68.78%
Nickel	:	0.52%
Methylamine	:	5.70
Reaction Pressure	:	2 - 2.5 Kg /cm^2
Temperature	:	15 - 20°C.
Agitation	:	200 RPM.

In the reactor vessel took first benzeen and then add to it phenylacetyl corbinol with agitation of 200RPM. After complete dissolution of phenylacetyl corbinol in benzeen added to the reactor requisite amount of methylamine to it and then added to it nickel as catalyst to the reactor. Make temperature of the reactor at 15 - 20°C and make pressure inside the reactor 2 - 2.25 kg /cm^2 compressed air. Reaction continued around 4 hours. After four hours took out the sample and check wheather ephidrine has formed or not. Took out the reacted liquid containing ephidrine is decant out or filter out to seperate catalyst.

Add concentrated hydrocholric acid to the nide free reacted liquid. After adition of hydro chloric acid reacted liquid is washed by action, two loyers formed, tool out lower layers, now cower layers be Concentrated by vaccumevaporator and child it to 5 - 10° C for form ephidrine hydrocholoride crustal, seperate it by contrifugation method or filtration method.

Now prepared crystal pack and market it.

Manufacturing Process Flow Diagram

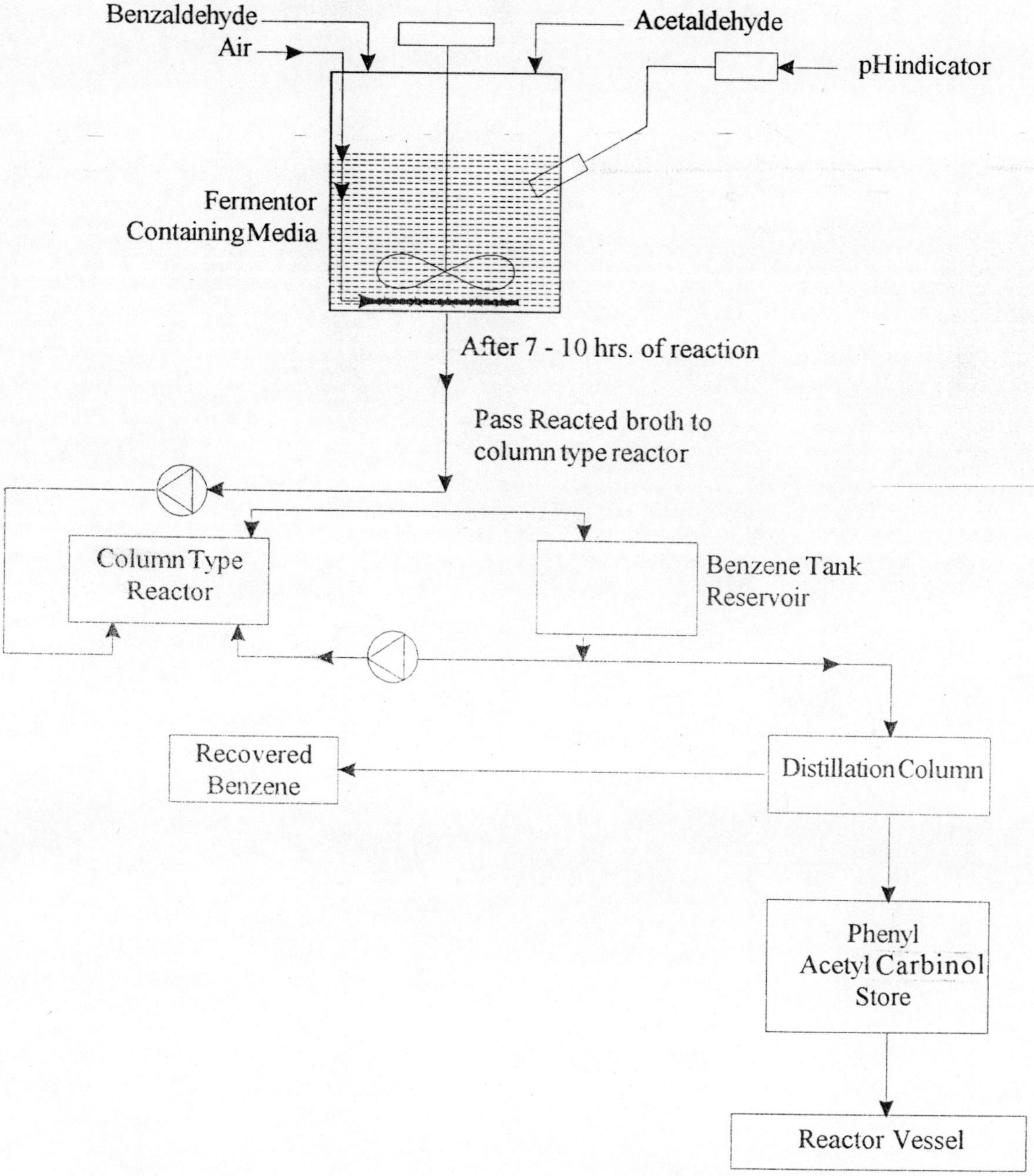

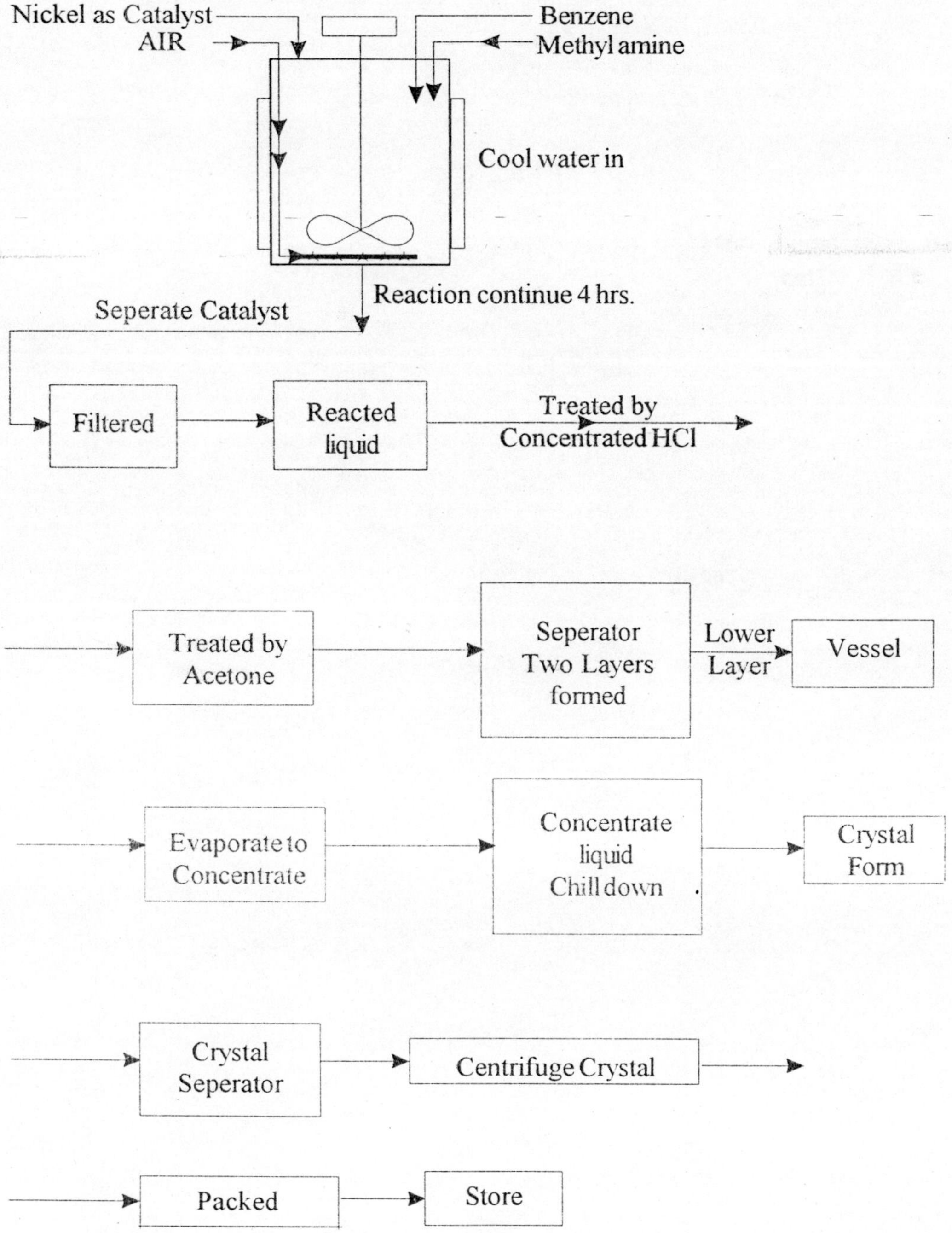
Nickel as Catalyst
AIR
Benzene
Methyl amine
Cool water in
Reaction continue 4 hrs.
Seperate Catalyst
Filtered
Reacted liquid
Treated by Concentrated HCl
Treated by Acetone
Seperator Two Layers formed
Lower Layer
Vessel
Evaporate to Concentrate
Concentrate liquid Chill down
Crystal Form
Crystal Seperator
Centrifuge Crystal
Packed
Store

Anhydrous Ephedrine :

Properties

Colourless crystals or white crystaline powder, odourless or with a slight aromatic odour. It rapidly absorbs carbondioxide, melting point about 38°C.

Solubilities

1 in 20 of water very Soluble in alcohol, soluble in CH Cl_3, ether, glycerol, olive oil and liquid paraffin solution in water are strongly alkaline to items. Solutions in oil are free from turbidity. Ephedrine decompose on exposure to light. Store in cool place in air tight container. Protect from light.

Uses

Anhydrous ephedrine has been used for preparing oil solution of ephedrine.

Ephidrine Hydrochloride

L. Ephidrine Hydrochlorium ($C_{10}H_{15}NO$, HCl - 201.7)

Dose

15 - 60 mg, I.P, max - in 24 Hours. 150 mg by mouth, 120 mg substaneously.

Odourless, colourless crystals or white crystaline powder with a bitter, taste, M.Pt. 217 °C - 220°C.

Solubility

1 in 4 Water, 1 in 17 of Alcohol and 1 in 60 of glycerol. Practically insoluble in $CHcl_3$ and ether. In soluble in olive oil and liquid paraffin. A 3.2% Solution in water is isosmeric with Serum solution and sterilised by Auto doing or by filtration. Store in airtight container. Protect from light.

Production of 6 A.P.A. (6 - aminopenicillanic Acid)

Basic Raw Materials :

(1) Penecillin G or Penecillin V

(2) Enzyme Bacterial Acylase or Fungal acylase.

(3) Acetone or Methylene chloride.

Manufacturing Process

Penecillin G Dissolve in acetone or methylenechloride to make pH - 8 by addition of very slowly caustic soda solution with continuous agitation at temp 25° - 30°C. Prepared this solution circulate this through the imobilised enzyme bacterial acylase matrial column at 35° - 40°C, pH -8 continously till Penecillin G converted to 6 - Amitopenicillanic Acid and produce phenyl Acetic Acid.

In case of use Penecillin use fungal Acylase (enzyme) as enzyme and pH of the solution maintained 10 at 50°C to produced 6APA.

[In case of acidic pH reverse reaction accurs].

$$\textit{Penicillin G + Bacterial} \xrightarrow[\text{Temp 35°C-40°C}]{\text{pH-8}}$$

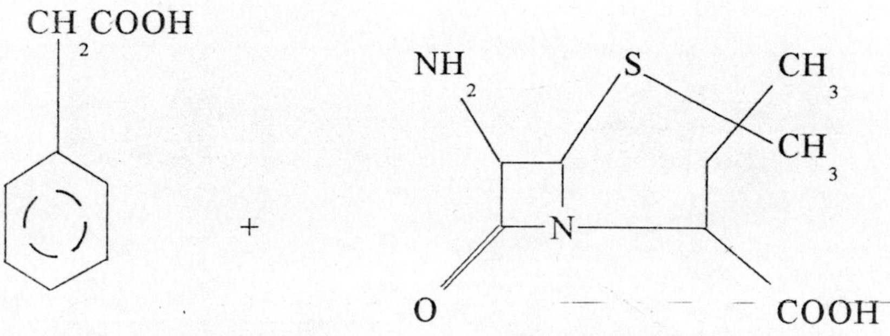

Phenyl Acetic Acid

6 Amino Penicillinic

Mixed reacted solution contains 6 APA and phenylacetic Acid pass through centrifugation, vacuum distillation and lastly by freeze drying process to get 6APA crystal.

USES

6 APA

6APA is the raw material for semisynthetic penicillins namely Ampicillin, Amoxycillin, Cloxacillin, Epicillin etc.

Trimethprime

Manufacturing Process

Basic Raw Materials required :

1. Ethyl cyanide.
2. Dimethyl ether.
3. Trimethoxy Benzaldehyde.
4. Guanidine.
5. Sulfuric Acid.

Ethylcyanide dissolve in dimethyl ether or ethylcyanide dissolve in ethyl alcohol in presence of glacial acetic acid took in a reactor to reflux at 110° - 120°C for 2 Hrs - 3 Hrs to convert ethyl cyanide to *b*-methoxy ethyl cyanide.

$$C_2H_5CN + CH_3OCH_3 \xrightarrow[\text{at Temp. } 110^{\circ}C-120^{\circ}C]{\text{Refulx 2-3 Hours}}$$

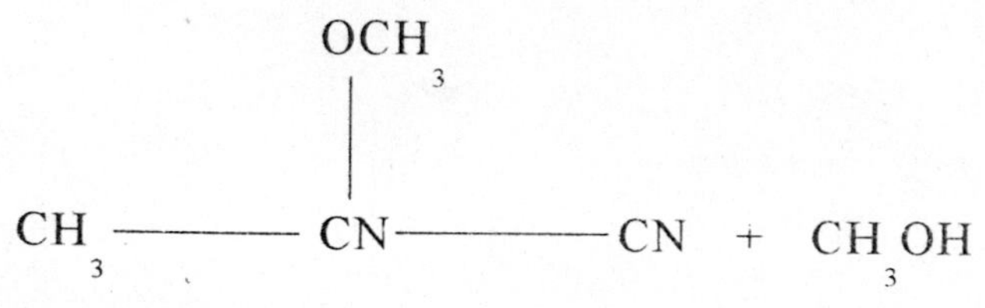

After completion of the reaction, add trimethoxy benzaldehyde to it make it alkaline by addition of caustic solution to make pH - 12 - 14, reflux alkaline Solution at 140^{0} C for 4 - 6 Hrs, by refluxation 3, 4, 5 trimethoxy benzaldehyde convert to 3, 4, 5 trimethoxy 2 cyano-dihydrocina maldehyde and methyl alcohol.

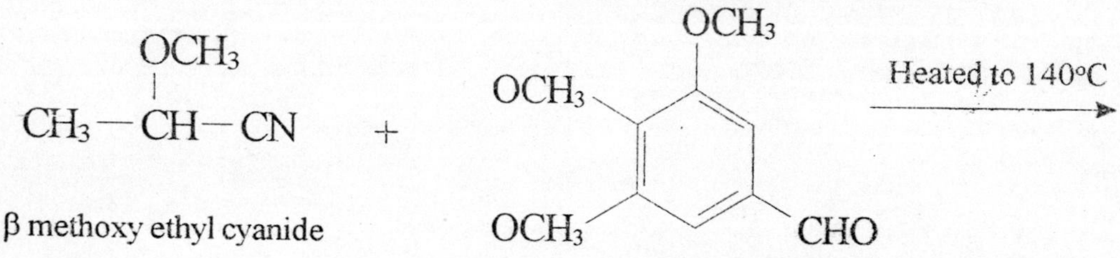

β methoxy ethyl cyanide

3,4,5 Trimethoxy Benzaldehyde

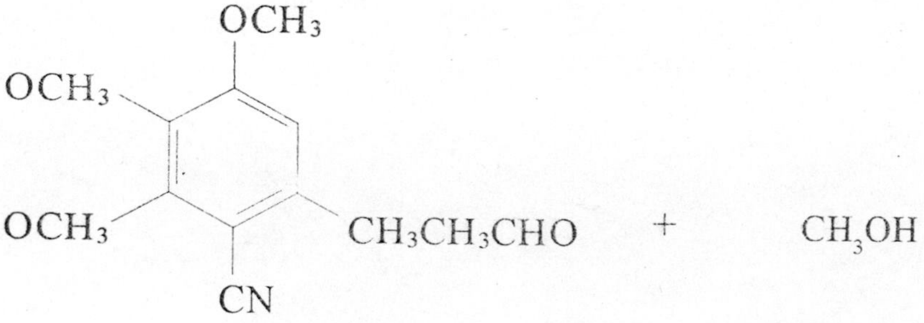

3,4,5 Trimethoxy
2 Cyanodihydrocinnamaldihyde

Methyl Alcohol

Now formed 3, 4, 5, Trimethoxy 2 cyanodilhydro cinnamaldehyde and methyl alchohol mixed with glacial acetic acid heated to 110°C - 125°C about 2 Hrs to form 3, 41 51 trimethoxy cyanodihydro cinnamaldehyde dimethyl acetal crystal

Dissolve 3, 4, 51 trimethoxy cyanodihydro cinnamaldehyde dimethyl acutal crystal in methyl alcohol and mixed with guanidine in the reactor vessel,heated to 123°C for 6 Hrs. to form trmethprime.

3, 4, 5, Trimethoxy xyanodihydro cinnamaldehyde dimethyl + Guanidine Acetal

Heated to 120°C →

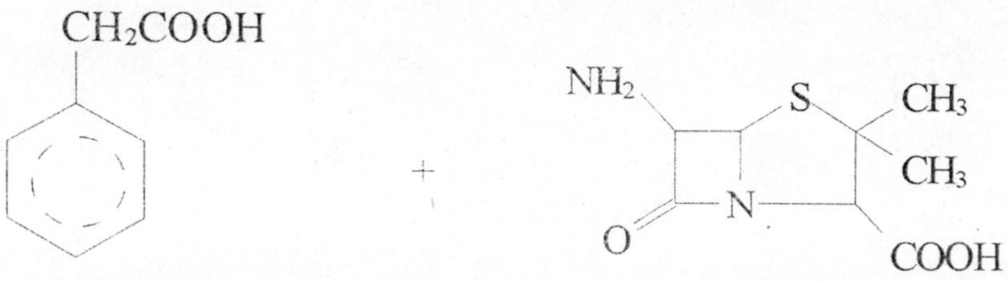

Phenyl Acetic Acid 6 Amino Penicillinic Acid

When trimethoprime is treated with concentrated sulfuric acid it forms trimethoprime sulfate. It forms coloured solution in water. For removal of Colour, the solution is treated by approximately 0. 2% of activated carbon on the wt. basis of trimethoprime sulfate salt at 40°C -50°C for 1/2 an hour. After carbon treatment solution filtered to seperate carbon free clear trimethoprime solution cool it and crystalise it to get clear colourless crystal from 90% concentrated solution. Now to get solution salt of trimethoprime solution is treated by caustic solution to form sodium salt of trimethoprime crystal.

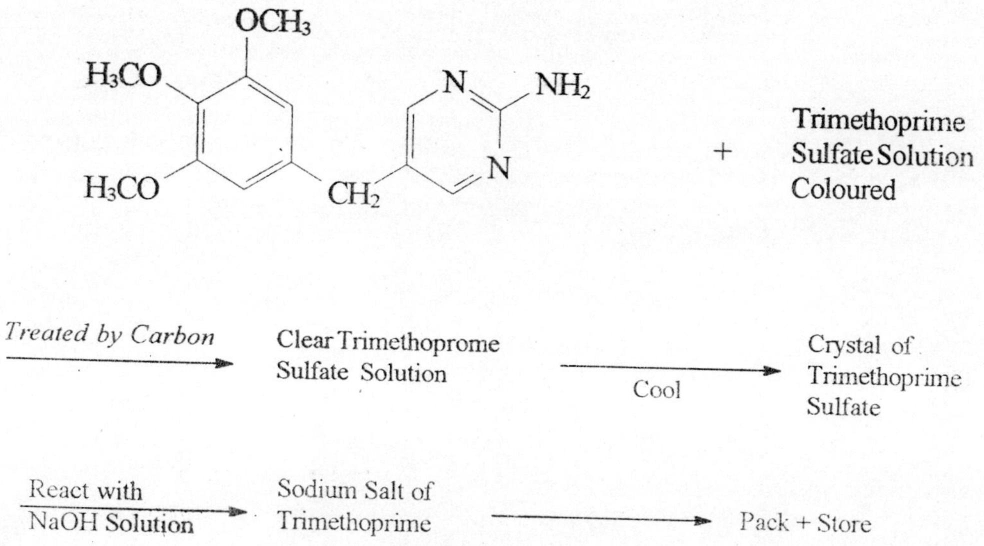

D - Phenyl glycinchloride Hydrochloride

Manufacturing Process

Basic Raw Materials are :

1. Benzaldehyde.
2. Potassium Cyanide.
3. Ammonia.
4. Ammonium Chloride.
5. Tartaric Acid
6. Hydrochloric Acid
7. Acetic Acid.

Well closed properly designed reactor in which cool liquor of ammonia and ammonium chloride are added to Benzaldehyde with constant stirring at temperature 35°C to maintain pH 14. It should be properly take care that there is no leakage in the reactor. After complete mixing of benezaldehyde, added requisite quantity of potassium cyanide very carefully to the reactor in highly alkaline medium of pH - 14 Now forms intermediate compound of benzaldehyde cyanohydrine compound which is further converted to 1 amino cyano Benzaldehyde in presence of excess liquor ammonia at pH 12 -14 temparature 35°C.

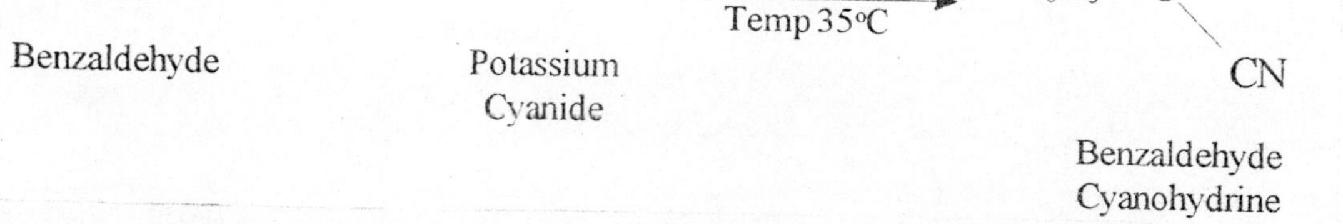

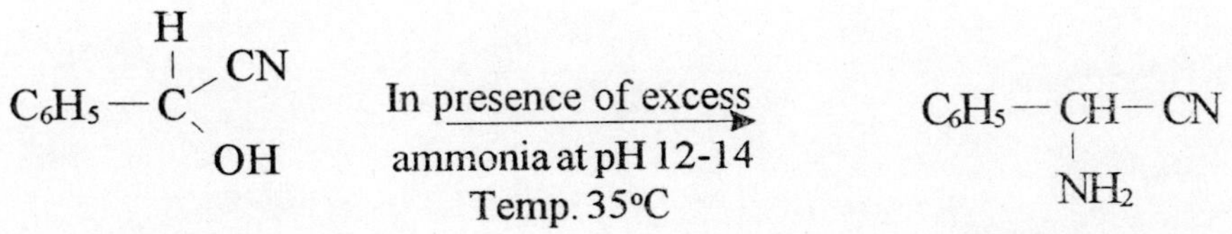

1 amonia cyano
Benzaldehyde

Added in this intermediate mixture excess quantity of tartaric acid solution at 40 - 45°C with continuous agitation to form D- Phenyl glycin, After complete formation of D- Phenyl glycin it is extract out by ethylene dichloride solvent. By complete agitation and mixing keep the mixture for one - two hours such that two layers will be separate out one aqueous layer and other organic solvent (ethylene dichloride layer) layer. Organic solvent layer contains D- Phenyl glycin chloride and aqueous layer contain tartaric acid.

Now organic layer ethylenedichloride distilled out and residue obtained D- phenyl glycin chloride crystal. Now treat concentrated Hydrochloric acid to get D- Phenyglycin chloride hydrochloride crystal.

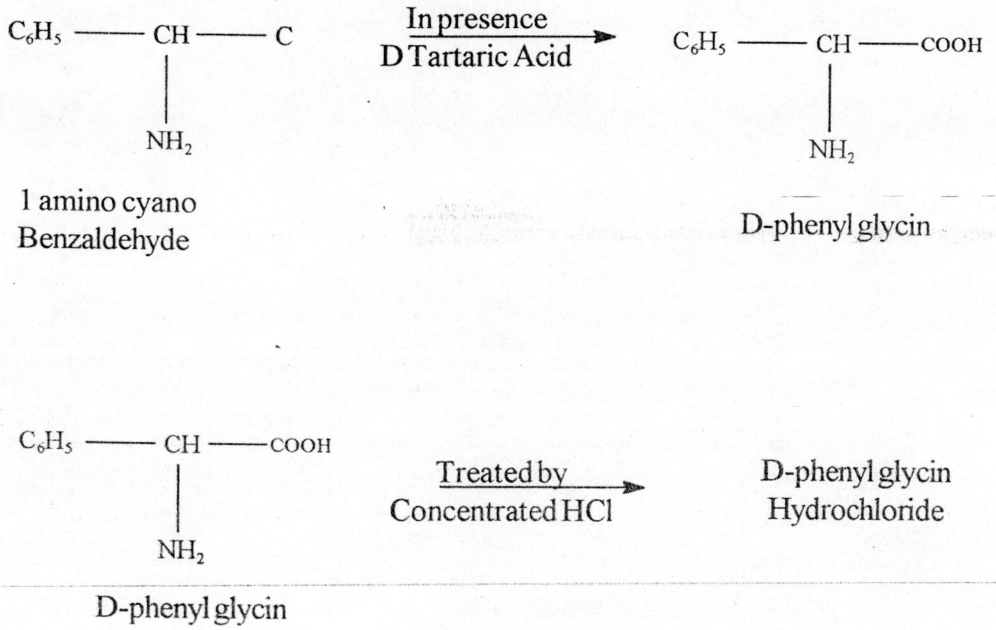

Aqueous layer contains tartaric acid. Add lime solution to tartaric acid solution make pH 5.5 at 60° - $70^{O}C$ to get calcium tartarate ppt. Filter out to get calcium tartarate precipitate. Now sulfuric acid added to the calcium tartarate precipitate to form tartaric acid, pH 0.85-0.90. Evaporate this tartaric acid solution at $60^{O}C$ - $70^{O}C$ at 550 - 600 mm. vacuum.

When concentration of the tartaric Acid solution becomes 90 - 95%, keep the solution for crystalisation at $20^{O}C$ - $15^{O}C$. Crystals are separate out by centrifuge process. It requires to dry the crystal at $35^{O}C$ - $40^{O}C$.

Process Flow Diagram

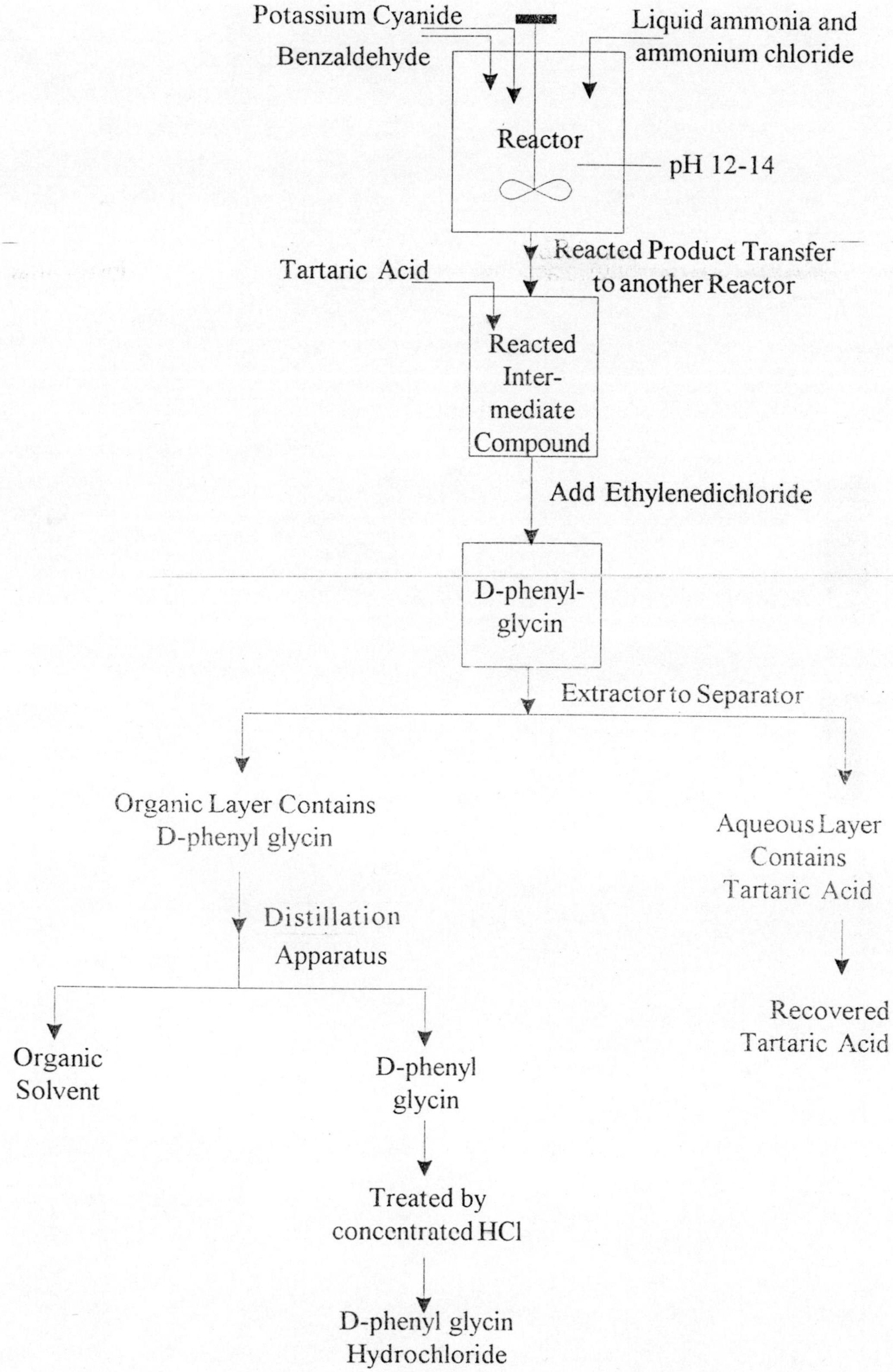

Uses

D - Phenylglycin or it's hydrochloride salps are largely used as intermediate product of in the preparation of drugs as ampicillin and amoxycillin.

Properties

D-phenyl glycin ⟶

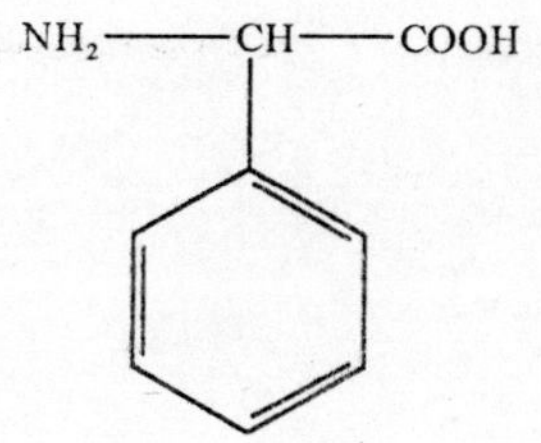

Molecular wt = 151

It is crystaline powder of melting point 245 - 248°C.

Solubility : Insoluble in water ether and ethanol.

Soluble in acid.

Preservation

Majority Drug or drug intermediate should be packed in clean packaging compound microbes free) and stored in clean low humid place at low terperature.

Temperature generally below 15°C.

Deoxribonuclic Acid (DNA)

Manufacturing Process : Deoxribonuclic Acid (DNA) from sheep-liver.

Basic Raw Materials are

1. Sheep liver.

2. Hydrochloric Acid.

3. Buffer solution of Sodium chloride and disodium salt of EDTA.

4. Sodium Lauryl Sulphate Solution.

5. Chloroform ; isopropanol and phenol.

6. Ribonuclease.

7. Phosphate buffer Containing cysteine hydrochloride, disodium salt of EDTA and crystalline papain.

8. Sodium acetate.

9. Ethanol.

10. Diethyl ether.

General Method of preparation

Sheepliver has been used as a starting material for the isolation of DNA. It is Commonly available in any Slaughter house. This material could be stored on ice for few hours before processing without any detectable damage to DNA.

The Solvents and the buffers used in various steps for the isolation of DNA.

S.No.	Steps	Solvent/Buffers used.
1.	Extraction : Homogenisation of liver	HCL Buffer Containing Sodium Chloride and Disodium Salt of EDTA.
2.	Lysing cells	Sodium lauryl Sulfate Solution.
3.	Denaturation and Coagulation of proteins.	A mixture of $CHcl_3$ isopropanol and phenol. (All Solvents Should be distilled before use)
4.	Dissolution of DNA	A dilute Solution of sodium salt of EDTA.
5.	Ribonuclease Treatment	A dilute solution of disodium salt of EDTA containing an appropriate amount RNA ase.

6.	Deproteinisation	A Phosphate buffer containing cystein Hcl, disodium salt of EDTA and appropriate amount of crystaline papain.
7.	Precipitation of DNA as sodium salt	Sodium Acetate Solution and ethanol.
8.	Washing precipitated DNA	Washed by ethanol and Diethyl ether.

Extraction of DNA

Ship liver is homogenize by a Suitable homogenizer by using Suitable buffer Solution which will produce thin cell Suspension. Now this solution is pass through the filtration to separate fibers from the cells. The separated cells are now loses by using Sodium lauryl Sulfate Solution. Now add phenol to the Solution or phenol and Chloroform mixture in the Solution and heat it to coagulate and precipitated out of protein. Centrifuge the Solution to take out ppt and got the centrifuge liquid. Wash the ppt by disodium salt of EDTA to dissolve DNA and collect it and mixed it with centrifuge liquid, completly deproteinized this liquid by using buffer Solution containing cystein hydrochloride, disodium salt of EDTA and appropriate amount of crystaline papain. Separate out the precipitate by centrifuging and collect centrifuged liquid. Now DNA has been precipitated out from the solution by addition of sodium acetate solution and ethanol. Now again by centrifugation to separate out DNA.

Finally, the DNA is Washed, dried and stored in vacuum desicator at $40^{\circ}C$ free from moisture.

1gm DNA produced from 1 kg sheepliver.

Specifications of sheepliver DNA

Deoxyribose Content	:	45 ± 2%
Phosphorus	:	9.2 ± 0.2%
Protein	:	4 ± 1%
Averag Molecular wt	:	5.8×10^6.
Molecular Wt. Coefficient		
(S_2O)	:	19.2 ± 1.45[5]

Structure of DNA

Deoxyribonucleic acid or (DNA) is the nucleic acid that accurs in combination with protein in the chromosomes and contains genetic instructions. It consists of four primary nitrogenous base (adenine, guanaine, thymine, cytosine), and phosphoric acid arranaged in a regular structure. The skeleton of the DNA Consists of two chains of alternate sugar and phosphate groups, twisted around each other in the form of double spiral or double helix, to each sugar is attached above, and the two chains are held together by hydrogen bonding between the bonds.

The sequence of bases provides in code the genetic information, which is transcribed, edited and acted on the RNA. Each human cell nucleous contains approximately 6 X 10 base pairs of DNA.

Brief Analysis of India's Export of Pharmaceutical Products to EU During 1993 over all export of pharmaceutical products from Extra. EU Countries to EU.

During 1993, a total quantity of 95884 tons of pharmaceutical products valued at ECU 5442.8 million was exported from extra - EU Countries to EU, which accounted for 1.12 percent by value of the total export of all products (ECU 485. 93 billion) from extra EU Countries to EU during the same period. Export of pharmaceutical products from extra EU Countries to EU has increased by 12.17% in value during 1993 over the previous year. (Table 1) and between 1988 and 1993 exports from Extra - EU Sources to EU have grown by about 140% i.e. at an average rate of 23% per year (Table 2).

In previous years, the pharmaceutical giants such as switzerland, U.S.A, Sweeden, Austria, and Japan continued to dominate the European pharmaceutical market during the period under review, Together, these five Countries accounted for over 91.01% of the total extra - EU. export of pharmaceutical to EU in 1993 (Table 3).

Among the EU 12, Germany is thetop most importer of pharmaceutical products accounting for 26.8% of the total import from extra - EU Countries in 1993, followed by France (15.7%), Italy (15.4%), UK (14.8%) Belgium - Luxemburg (7.2%), The Netherland, (6.6%), Spain (5.8%) etc.

India shipped out 773 tons of pharmaceutical products valued at ECU 7.33 million to EU in 1993, which accounted for only 0.13% of the total extra - EU export of pharmaceuticals to EU during the same period. In 1993 India ranked seventeenth among the principal extra. EU exporters of pharmaceuticals to EU after South Korea, Developing Countries Such as China, Brazil, Argentina, Israel, Poland, Hungary and South Korea had a better store in the EU market for pharmaceuticals then that of India during the year 1993 (Table 1)

Export of pharmaceutical products from India to EU, which has been increasing steadily at an average rate of 32 % per year between 1988 - 1992 has decreased by 28.46% in 1993. (from ECU 10.24 million in 1992 to ECU 7.23 million in 1993) over the previous year, (Table 1 and 2).

UK is the top most importer of pharmaceutical products from India accounting for 49.9% of our total exports to EU in 1993 followed by Belgium Luxemburg (30.6%), Germany (12.7%), Italy (2.8%) etc. Together, these four Countries accounted for 96% of our total export of pharmaceuticals to EU during 1993. (Table 1).

Principal Items Export

Principal Items of pharmaceutical products exported from Extra- EU Countries as well as India to EU during 1993 are shown in (Table - 3).

Medicoments falling under CN. Code No. 3004 were the main items of export from India to EU during 1993 and these items accounted for over 72.7% of the total export of pharmaceuticals from India to EU., followed by items falling under on Code No. 3005 (13.4%) and items under on code No 3003 (10.0%) while export of items falling under CN. Code 3005 has gone up by 71.8% in 1993 over the previous year, export of items falling under CN. Code Nos. 3003 and 3004 have decreased by 71.3% and 16.7% respectively during the some period.

Considering, the importance of pharmaceutical products falling under on Code Nos 3004, 3005, and 3003 which Constitute bulk of our export to EU, India's Export of the above products to EU vis a vis extra EU are analysed below in greater detail.

Export of pharmaceutical products falling under CN. Code No 3004.

The main items of pharmaceutical products falling under C.N. Code No. 3004 are as follows.

Medicoments (excluding goods of C.N. Code No. 3002, 3005, 3006). Consisting of mixed or unmixed products for therapeatic or prophylaetic uses, put up in measured does or packaging for retail sale and containing penicillin, other antibiotics harmones such as insulin, adrenal cortical harmones and others.

During 1993 the above items worth ECU 3627.3 million were exported from Extra EU Countries to EU. Switzerland was the top most exporter accounting 50.5% of the total Extra - EU Export in 1993. India ranked 12th among the principal extra EU Exporters of these itemes to EU in 1992 and it's share in total Extra - EU export was 0. 16%.

Important items of products and CN. Code NO - 3004 Exported from India to EU during 1993 are shown in Table -2.

Export of pharmaceutical Products falling under **CN. Code No. -3005**.

Wadding, gaetze, bandages and similar articles, impregnated or couted with pharmaceutical substones are the important items falling under the U.N. Codes NO - 3005.

India's export of the above items to EU, which has been decreasing steadily from 1988 - 1992, has picked up again by 71.88% in 1993, over the previous year, However, the export of 0.93 million E.C.U. in 1993 is less than the record maximum export of 1.25 million E.C.U in 1988. U.K. is the major importer of these items from India followed by Italy.

Export of pharmaceutical Products falling under C.N. Code No 3003.

Medicanents (excluding good f cw. Code nos 3002, 3005 or 3006) Consisting of two or more constituents which have been mixed together and containing penecillins, other antibiotics insulin, alkaloids and other item falling under the CW. Code NO - 3003.

India export was only 0.75 million ECU during 1993. while export of above items from extra - EU to EU has increased by 4. 18% in 1993 over the previous year.

Ref.

India Trade Centre.

Bru scales (Belgium)

Brief Analysis of Indian Export during 1993 for

(1) Agriculture pro.

(2) Pharmaceutica!

(3) Marine Products.

Con. codes Country NameCOMPLITIOR ANALYSIS TABLE -1
PRODUCT-WISE EEC EMPORTOTT : MT
DURING JAN- DEC. 1993 VALUE : 000 ECU

PAGE SHARE w.r.t. VALUE
PROD-CODE : 30

PRODUCT : Pharmacuetical products
TOTAL IMPORTS

CON. CODES	COUNTRY	NAME	EEC (12)	FRANCE	BEL-LUX	NETHRL	FRG.	ITALY	U.K.	IRELAND	DENMARK	GREECE	PORTGL	SPAIN.
1011	EXTRA-EC	QTY.	95884	13971	5752	6003	30024	18159	12106	777	3596	1810	850	2836
		VALUE	5442805	856377	394224	6003	1460200	840503	805029	37681	166673	126339	83039	313689
	sage	SHARE	100.00	-----	-----	-----	-------	-------	------	------	-------	-------	------	---------
36	SWITTZERLAND	QTY.	27060	3553	2939	1933	11263	2502	2492	58	234	967	560	559
		VALUE	2185098	378703	245777	115858	43858	480163	243985	1587	28549	84948	62534	110791
	sage	SHARE	40.15	44.22	62.34	32.45	29.59	57.13	30.23	4.21	17.13	67.24	75.24	35.32
400	UNITED STATES	QTY.	15201	1359	579	2339	4144	1460	3590	293	325	280	67	765
		VALUE	1307631	157545	73744	101632	463829	156518	201222	19489	25970	13457	5601	88560
	sage	SHARE	24.03	18.40	18.71	28.48	31.76	18.62	24.93	51.72	15.58	10.66	6.75	28.23.
30	SWEDEN	QTY.	9896	2323	446	662	1616	487	1632	9	2033	235	64	336
		VALUE	990160	182037	26116	94651	232637	33093	232902	146	84652	19994	9185	73745
	sage	SHAME	13.19	21.26	6.62	25.51	15.00	3.94	23.85	0.33	50.79	15.83	11.05	23.51
38	AUSTRIA	QTY	22601	3718	152	150	7304	9762	202	268	20	62	87	371
		VALUE	348017	20839	22768	21445	1706934	77798	11610	7815	1794	1612	2567	9025
	sage	SHARE	6.39	2.44	5.78	6.01	11.69	9.25	1.44	20.4	1.08	1.28	3.09	2.83
732	JAPAN	QTY.	731	125	146	14	135	101	150	11	10	8	5	25
		VALUE	136422	47249	5682	2684	30676	28365	7056	3281	1896	881	318	8334
	sage	SHARE	2.51	5.52	1.44	0.75	2.10	3.37	0.87	8.71	1.14	0.70	0.38	2.66

404	CANADA	QTY.	2004	514	32	54	340	487	465	23	14	4	9	56
		VALUE	68427	3677	1269	760	31812	9268	15468	2113	1111	372	480	2097
	sage	SHARE	1.26	0.43	0.32	0.21	2.81	1.10	1.92	5.61	0.67	0.29	0.58	0.67
32	FINLAND	QTY.	939	30	232	176	175	6	97	5	201	0	0	17
		VALUE	62396	12251	3662	2520	15664	1108	19081	270	6997	216	8	619
	sage	SHARE	1.15	1.43	0.93	0.71	1.07	0.13	2.36	0.72	4.20	0.17	0.01	0.20
28	NORWAY	QTY.	2479	381	48	32	1371	9	302	35	288	8	0	5
		VALUE	62214	19054	3379	2589	7321	883	13227	1839	11609	1672	16	625
	sage	SHARE	1.14	2.22	0.86	0.73	0.50	0.11	1.64	4.88	6.97	1.32	0.02	0.20
800	AUSTRALIA	QTY.	1063	18	3	58	20	2	942	8	0	2	9	1
		VALUE	53728	15208	141	4808	4448	109	27691	243	194	190	638	52
	sage	SHARE	0.99	1.78	0.04	1.35	0.30	0.01	3.34	0.6	0.12	0.15	0.77	0.02

SOURCE : CUROSTAT

Selection Critria for Competitors : EX-EC. India & Top n

INDIA TRADE CENTRE
BRUSSLESS. BELGIUM.

COMELITORS ANALYSIS
PRODUCT.i-WISE EEC EMPORT TABLE - 1
DURING Jan-Dec.1993 QTY. : MI
VALUE: 000 ECU
Sage SHARE w.r.t. VALUE

PROD-CODE :30
PRODUCT : Pharmaceutical Products
TOTAL IMPORTS

CON CODES	COUNTRY	NAME	EEC(12)	FRANCE	BEL-LUX	NETHRL.	FRG.	ITALY	U.K	IRELAND	DENMARK	GREECE	PORTGL	SPAIN
720	CHINA	QTY.	7069	843	703	34	1274	2113	1143	8	300	87	13	533
		VALUE	42223	4338	4296	186	15989	7435	3265	130	1506	928	89	4061
	sage	SHARE	0.78	0.51	1.09	0.05	1.09	0.88	0.40	0.35	0.90	0.73	0.11	1.29
508	BRAZIL	QTY.	184	34	1	3	8	124	9	1	0	2	2	0
		VALUE	23252	1193	97	72	7281	13066	1300	6	0	54	103	80
	sage	SHARE	0.43	0.14	0.02	0.02	0.15	1.55	0.16	0.02	0.00	0.04	0.12	0.03
528	ARGENTINA	QTY.	153	40	41	0	17	39	1	0	11	0	0	4
		VALUE	17058	2698	83	0	271	5449	122	20	36	0	25	8354
	sage	SHARE	0.31	0.32	0.02	0.00	0.02	0.65	0.02	0.05	0.02	0.00	0.03	2.66
624	ISRAEL	QTY.	255	34	22	6	94	20	37	0	1	22	2	17
		VALUE	13656	1807	433	1218	6287	1053	1459	7	42	219	100	1031
	sage	SHARE	0.25	0.21	0.11	0.34	0.43	0.13	0.18	0.02	0.03	0.17	0.12	0.33
60	POLAND	QTY.	365	99	5	29	148	13	36	0	35	0	0	0
		VALUE	12899	721	259	301	4284	777	6035	0	462	0	0	0
	sage	SHARE	0.24	0.08	0.07	0.08	0.29	0.09	0.76	0.00	0.28	0.00	0.00	0.00
64	HUNGARY	QTY.	343	32	2	21	127	137	7	0	2	6	8	1
		VALUE	12403	765	93	149	7898	680	1535	0	68	823	382	10
	sage	SHARE	0.23	0.09	0.02	0.04	0.54	0.08	0.19	0.00	0.04	0.65	0.46	0.00

728	KOREA DEM.REP	QTY.	183	2	25	83	2	19	39	0	6	0	5	2
		VALUE	7471	146	845	400	524	2892	1380	0	1023	56	157	48
	sage	SHARE	0.14	0.02	0.21	0.11	0.04	0.34	0.17	0.00	0.61	0.4	0.19	0.02
664	INDIA	QTY.	773	6	233	3	107	82	335	1	0	6	0	0
		VALUE	7329	47	2245	140	931	203	3657	46	1	58	0	1
	sage	SHARE	0.13	0.01	0.5777	0.04	0.06	0.02	0.45	0.12	0.00	0.05	0.00	0.00

SOURCE : EUROSTAT   Selection Critria for Competitors : EX-EC. India & Top n   228/1994   1:44:1   INDIA TRADE CENTER BRUSSLES, BELGIUM

SOURCE : EUROSTAT   Selection Critria for Competitors :EX-EC.India & Top n   INDIA TRADE CENTER BRUSSLES, BELGIUM

TABLE - 2

EU Imports From Extra - EU
Product : 30

1988	1988	1989	1990	1991	1992	1993
EXTRA-EC	2272536	2780841	3329267	4031241	4852357	5442806
		22. 37%	19.72%	21.08%	20.37%	12.17%
SWITZERLAND	1068602	1249571	154675	1823101	2020978	2185098
		16.94%	23.78%	17.87%	10.85%	8.12%
USA	438388	594158	681514	841040	1111574	1307637
		35.53%	14.70%	23.41%	32.17%	17.64%
SWEDEN	341148	439033	519770	668978	868366	990160
		28.69%	18.39%	28.71%	29.80%	14.03%
AUSTRIA	194848	227795	241928	265811	318842	348017
		16.91%	6.20%	9.87%	19.95%	9.15%
JAPAN	29957	41499	52812	94331	125049	136422
		38.53%	51.35%	50.13%	32.56%	9.09%
CANADA	16647	26439	44958	49973	45065	63427
		58.82%	70.04%	11.15%	-9.82%	51.84%
INDIA	3500	3853	4667	7084	10244	7329
		10.09%	21.13%	51.79%	44.61%	-28.45%

TABLE - 3

	Total Extra-EU export to EU	Total India's export to EUEU	Percentage Share in the total extra export to		Main extra-EU exporters and EU by value their share	
	Qty	Val.	Qty	Val.		
Pharmaceutical Products Total	95884	5442.8	773	7.330.13	Switzerlanl	40.2%
					USA	24.0%
					Swden	18.2%
					Austria	6.4%
!. Items of CN Code No.3001 :	937	178.9	-	-	Switzerland	31.5%
Lands & organs dride, extracts of					USA	302%
lands & organs, haparin & its salts					Sweden	8.3%
etc for organs- therapaitoc uses					China	6.2%
2. Items of CN Code No. 3002 :	17236	1078.2	-	0.02	USA	57%
moon blod, animal blood prepared					Austria	19.2%
for therapautic, prophylactic and					Swizerland	15.8%
stagnostic uses, vaccines for human					Canada	2.0%
and veterinary medicines, etc.						
3. Items of CN Code No. 3003 :	6708	320.7	101 0.75	0.23	Swizerland	34.6%
Redicaments (excl. SL. Nos 2,5&6)					Sweden	18.9%
of two more constituents for					USA	12.9%
therapautic and prophylatic uses-					Austria	10.0%
containing antibiotics, alkolaids,					Japan	9.2%
fodine compounds, etc.					Canada	6.5%
4. Items of CN Code No. 3004 :	48614	3267.3	423	5.33	0.16	
Redicaments (excl. SL No. 2,5 & 6)					Switzerland	50.5%
of aixed/unmixed products for					Sweden	27.2%
therepautic/prophylactic uses-					USA	11.6%
containing penicillin, other anti-					Japan	2.3%
biotics, hormones, Vitamins,					Austria	2.1%
alkaloids etc.						
5. Items of CN Code No 3005 : 18968	376.2	228	0.98	0.26	Switzerland	39.9%
Wedding, gauze, bandages, impregnated					USA	38.1%
or coated with pharmaceuticals,					China	6.9%
substances for medical, surgical,					Austria	3.9%
dental or veterinary purposes					Sweden	2.7%
6. Items of CN Code No 3006 :	3421	221.1	21	0.05		
Pharmaceutical goods such as surgical					USA	34.3%
cetgut, sterile laminaria, dental					Switzerland	21.8%
haemostatics, dental cement, first					Norway	16.6%
aid boxes, chemical contraceptive					Austria	7.9%
preparations etc.					Sweden.	4.0%

Following machineries are required generally in any pharmaceutical bulk drug industry.

1. Reaction vessels : With hot and cold water circulation provision. Designer will consider the material of construction.(Material generally used SS - 304, 55 - 316, SS316 L or M.S. with lining of glass or rubber).
2. Crystalliser.
3. S.S.Tank or P.P.Tank.
4. Refrigeration unit.
5. Centrifugation unit : It may be bucket type or high speed disc bowl or Nozzle type centrifuge.
6. Filtration unit : It may nutche type filter, drum filters, plate and frame filter etc.
7. Vacuum pump.
8. S.S. Pipes, G.I. pipes, or P.P. pipes.
9. Deminerelising unit.
10. Motors, Starters.
11. Boiler.
12. Drier.
13. Cooling Tower.

Address of Plant and Machinery Suppliers

Reaction vessels

1. Buckau wolf India Ltd.

   Pimpri,

   Pune - 411018.

   India.

   Tel. : 84461.

2. Chemech Engineering

   106 Sharma Industrial Estate

   Walbat Road,

   Goregoan (East)

   Bombay - 400063.

   Phone : 691941.

3. Otoklin Plants and Equipment Ltd.

   1006 Prasad Chambers,

   Bombay - 400004.

   Tel. : 369372.

Centrifuge Machine

4. Benett and Company Ltd.

   P.O. Box. 46

   Aridover

   Hampshire

   Tel. : 0980 - 64488.

5. APTE Analgamations Ltd.

   4th floor, 199 Church gate,

   Reclamation.

   Bombay - 400020,

   India.

   Tel. : 091 - 22 - 2871194 / 95

   Telex : 011 - 83790 TECHIN

   Fax : 091 - 22 - 2871405

6. Alfa Laval India Ltd.

   DAPODI.

   PUNE - 411012

   INDIA.

   Tel. : 86321 (6lines)

Filtration unit

7. Filtech Pharmalab Pvt. Ltd.

   Star Metal Compound.

   L. B. S. Marg.

   Vikhroli (West)

   Bombay - 400083.

   India.

   Tel. : 091 - 22 - 5782559.

   Telex : 011 - 71934.

   Fax : 022 - 5785329.

8. SANTECH, USA

   RR Box. 799, Lata Yette

   N.J. 07848 - 9405 U.S.A.

   Fax : 201 - 579 - 1060

9. Toshniwal Brothers (Bombay) Pvt Ltd.

   198 Jamshedji Tata Road,

   Bombay - 400020,

   India.

   Tel. : 091 - 22 - 221565.

   Fax : 091 - 22 - 2040396.

Drier - Biotech

10. Spinco Biotech Private Ltd.

    35 Vaidy aram Street,

    T. Nagar,

    Madras : 600017,

    India.

    Tel. : 091 - 44 - 4340174.

    Fax : 091 - 044 - 4340761.

11. Arcting India Sales

    20 Rajpur Road,

    Delhi - 110054.

    Tel. : 2912800, 2522424,

    Fax : 91 - 11 - 2521754.

Refrigeration Machine

12. Blue Star Ltd,

    Band Box House, Prabhadevi,

    Bombay - 400025

    Telephone : 4933101

    Fax : 91 - 22 - 4933799.

Cooling Tower

13. Paharpur Cooling Towers P. Ltd.
8/1/B Diamond Harbour Road,
Calcutta - 700027.

Boiler

14. Thermax Limited.
4 Bombay Pune Road,
Shivaji nagar
Pune - 411005
Tel. : 0212 - 51123,
Fax : 0212 - 55041.

General Suppliers of Raw Materials

1. Biobusiness India Ltd.
C - 76, Fateh Nagar,
Jail Road,
New Delhi - 110018
India.
Tel. : 091 - 11 - 5596820
Fax : 091 - 11 - 5596820

2. International Solvents and
Chemical Company.
85 Nariana Bhawan,
Opposite Hoechst House,
227 Nariman Point.
Bombay - 400021,
Tel. : 2028162.

3. A. Choksey Chemicals Industries
101 M.G. Road Fort,
Bombay - 400023.
Tel. : 273868.

4. CHEM MART
51 /52 Shakhar Bhawan,
5th floor,
Nariman Point,
Bombay - 400021.
Phone : 2044563 /64.
Fax . 0222043971.

A

SELECTED PROJECTS FOR RIGHT INVESTMENT

- Watch Straps/Chains/Bracelets / Belt (Brass & Steel)
- Welding Brass Rod
- Welding Electrodes
- Welding Fluxes
- Wick Stoves
- Wick Stoves Stainless Steel
- Wind Mill
- Wind Screen Cleaner
- Wire Mesh (Hexagonal Square)
- Wire Nail
- Wire Nail/Wire Drawing
- Zinc And Aluminium Anode Foundry Marine & Oil Industry

Miscellaneous Products

- Advertising Agency
- Agarbatti (Sticks)
- Air Taxi (12 Seater)
- Amusement Park
- Amusement Park Cum Water Park
- Artificial Flowers (Paper & Cloth)
- Artificial Marble Tiles
- Asphlatic Roofing Sheet
- Auto Workshop/Garage & Service Station
- Bamboo Chips For Paper Mill
- Bamboo Sticks Used For Agarbatti
- Bamboo Tooth Picks (Cap. 64 Mt/Annum)
- Bank (Private Sector)
- Banquet Hall
- Batchlor Physiotherapy (BPT College).
- Bentonite (Quarrying, Processing & Exporting)
- Bone Crushing Plant
- Broom Stick Processing Unit.
- Buttons From Cattle Houses
- Buttons From Hoves & Horns
- Canvas Shoes
- Carbide Tips/Inserts/Indextable.
- Car-Leasing & Finance
- Cigarette
- Cigarettes Unit
- Cinema Hall
- Coal Washing Unit
- Coir Handicraft
- Coir Industries
- Cold Storage
- Cold Storage & Ice Plant
- Cold Storage (Cap. 6000 M.T)
- Combine Coke
- Community Hall
- Composite Carbon Fiber
- Cricket Ball, Bat Manufacturing
- Culinary Institute
- Daily Need Stores
- Dental Collage.
- Departmental Stores
- Diagnostic Centre
- Diamond & Gem Cutting & Processing Unit
- Diamond Cutting & Export
- Dispensary
- Disposable Cigarette Gas Lighter
- Dry Cleaners
- Dry Cleaning And Laundry Unit
- Dry Clock
- Dry Flowers
- Engineering College
- Expansion Joint Filler
- Eye Hospital
- Fast Food Corner
- Fire Fighting Equipment, Chemicals & Refilling
- Fire Works
- Five Star Hotel (Deluxe)
- Five Star Hotel Industry
- Five Star Hotels With (Shopping Mall, Health Club, Water Park, Amusement Park, Golf Course & Golf Academy, Cottage & Openair Theatre)
- Five Star Hotels, Business Center (Shopping Centre) PVR, Health Club & Banquet Hall
- Flush Door, Chip Board, Hard Board, Insulating Board
- Flush Door, Clip Board & Hardboard
- Games Parlour
- Gas Filling Of L.P.G. Cylinder
- Gems Manufacturing (Original)
- Gold & Silver Jewellery
- Gold Jewellery (100% Eou)
- Golf Course.
- Handicrafts (Can & Bamboo)
- Hard Board From Saw Dust
- Hawan Samgri
- Health Club & Beauty Parlour
- Health Club Cum Beauty Parlour Cum Hair Saloon
- Heat Chamber Painting
- Holiday Resorts
- Holiday Resorts Cum Entertainment Club 4 Star Hotel
- Holiday Village Resort
- Hospital
- Hospital (20 Beds)
- Hospital 300 Beds To 700 Beds Teaching Facility
- Hospital Bed
- Hotel
- Hotel 5 Star (Currency in Dollor).
- Hotel Industries 5 Star, 3 Star Holiday Resorts
- Hotel Unit (Three Star)
- Hotel/Small Motel
- International Standard laboratories.
- Kids Entertainment Cum Food Centre (Restaurant) At The Mfg. Mall
- L.P.G. Cylinder Retesting Unit
- L.P.G. Cylinder Testing Centre
- Laminated Partical Board
- Laundry
- Leasing Hire Purchase A/C
- Local Area Bank
- Low Ash Metallurgical Coke Plant.
- Marketing Arrangement And Distribution Strategy Of Wd-40
- Marketing Of Gram Shilps
- Match Box (Manual Process).
- Match Box Plant (Automatic)
- Medical College
- Medical College Hospital & Research Institute
- Melamine Crockery
- Metallurgical Coke Plant Cooking Coal.
- Mfg. Of Coloured Joint Filler Used For Jointing Tiles
- Mfg. Of Food Colour, Gms, Caramel, Reactive Dyes & Pigments
- Milk Powder, Pasteurised Milk, Butter, Cheese & Ghee
- Mineral Fillers For Application Paint, Paper, Rubber, Plastic
- Mineral Wool
- Motel/Small Hotel With Banquet Hall, Restaurant & Catering
- Multiplex Cinema Hall, PVR With Shopping Centre.
- Multistoried Commercial Complex
- Natural Care Centre
- Nursery School.
- Nursing Home
- Old Age Home, Orphan Children Hall & Dharamshala.
- Paint Brush
- Paint Driers
- Particle Board & Block Board With Sanding And Laminating
- Pediatric Hospital 25 Beds
- Petrol Pump
- Pharmaceutical Collage (B-Pharma & D-Pharma)
- Photo Lab. Cum Studio (100% Computerized)
- Plaster Of Paris Bandages
- Plywood
- Plywood & Plyboard
- Plywood (Phenol Bonded)
- Pre Laminated Particle Board.
- Puzzles.
- PVC Joint Fillings
- Q.S.S. Colour Lab.
- Quering Of Lime Stone
- Recreation And Health Club
- Rehabilitation Centre For Aged & Needy
- Residential Apartments
- Residential School (C.B.S.E. Pattern).
- Restaurant
- Restaurant/Fast Food Parlour
- Rock Wool Base Slag
- Rubber Wood Processing Plant
- Saw Mill
- School
- School (Secondary School).
- Shellac Manufacturing
- Shoe Uppers
- Slaughter House Beef Processing
- Slimming Centre & Health Club
- Snake Park
- Sport Shoe (Automatic Imported Plant)
- Sterilize Bone Meal
- Straw Board
- Stuff Toys
- Sunmica
- Super Market (Commercial Market)
- Synthetic Floating To Fishing Industry
- Synthetic Ruby and Sapphire
- Teak Wood & Meranti Doors –Solid & Semi-Solid Doors
- Tennis Ball
- Three Star Hotel (Comparative Market Survey Report Of Delhi & Kolkata)
- Timber (Wood) Seasoning
- Trading Business (Computer & Related Stationery)
- Trading Business (Rice, Salt, Dry Fruits Etc.)
- Trading Business (With Packaging Rice, Salt, Pulses, Etc)
- Travelling Agency
- Venetian Blind
- Video Film Studio
- Vocational Training Institutes.
- Ware House
- Water Park
- Wind Mill
- Wonder Fuel (Gel Type)
- Wood Wool Industry
- Wooden Chips For Supplying To Paper Mills
- Wooden Doors Windows Sheets TV Cabinet
- Wooden Furniture
- Wooden Furniture
- Wooden Furniture With Mediocre Automation
- Wooden Furniture With Seasoning Plant
- Wooden Needles For Tooth & Wooden Spoon For Ice Cream
- Wooden Tooth Pick
- Work Shop For Telco Truck

Leather & Leather Goods

- Leather Garments
- Leather Goods
- Leather Shoes
- Leather Shoes & Chappals
- Leather Shoes (Agra Type)
- Leather Straps For Wrist Watches
- Leather Tanning
- Leather Tanning (Goats &Cows)
- Shoe Uppers
- Sport Shoes (Automatic Imported Plant)

Oils & Fats

- Anilin Oil By Hydrogenation From Benzene
- Cardamom Oil
- Castor Oil (Batch Process)
- Castor Oil (Extraction & Refining)
- Castor Oil (Refining & Extraction)
- Castor Oil Derivative Oleo Resin
- Chilli Oil
- Coconut Oil From Copra
- Coconut Oil In Containers (Filtration & Airtight Packaging)
- Corn Oil (Maize Oil)
- Cotton Seed Oil
- Cotton Seed Oil (Extraction & Refined)
- Extraction Of Oil From Neem Seed
- Extraction Of Oil From Soyabean & Cotton Seed
- Extraction Of Oil From Tamarind Seed
- Extraction Of Sesame, Rice Bran & Palm Oil
- Fat Liquor (Sulfated Oil)
- Garlic Oil
- Ginger Oil
- Hydrogenation Of Non-Edible Oil
- Lemon Grass Oil
- Linseed Oil Manufacturing
- Maize Oil
- Margarine/Fat
- Mohwa Oil
- Neem Oil From Seeds
- Non-Formal Dye Fixing Oil
- Palm Oil
- Patchouli Oil
- Poppy Seed Oil By Expeller Process
- Poppy Seed Oil By Solvent Extraction Process
- Rainbow Colours On Metal
- Refined Oil (Cotton Seed Ground Nut Oil & Sunflower Oil
- Refined, Bleached, Palm Oil From Crude Palm Oil
- Rice Bran Extraction & Refining
- Rice Bran Oil
- Rubber Processing Oil
- Shesham Oil From Shesham Seed
- Shortening & Liquid Palm (Olien)
- Solvent Extraction Plant
- Sun Flower Seed Oil
- Tejpatta Oil From Tejpatta
- Turkey Red Oil
- Turpentine Oil And Rosin
- Virgin Coconut Oil
- Wheat Grem Oil
- Wool Batching Oil

Paper & Allied Products

- Absorbent Kraft Paper
- Amonia Paper
- Carbonless Paper.
- Card Board Boxes & Cartoons Of Paper
- Card/Gray Board From Pulp & Waste Paper
- Coated Paper & Board Art & Chrom
- Corrugated Board Box Plant (Printed & Laminated)
- Corrugated Sheet Board & Boxes
- Craft Paper & Special Paper
- Craft Paper From Waste Paper (Cap-15-2 TPD)
- Emery Sand Paper
- Exercise Note Book & Register
- Flute Paper From Waste Paper
- Hand Made Paper
- Hand Made Paper Using Recycled Hand Made Paper
- Hard Board From Baggase
- Kraft Paper & Mill Board From Waste Cartoon Boxes
- Kraft Paper From Waste Cartoon Boxes
- Manufacturing Of Recycled Paper Products
- Mini Paper Plant
- Mini Paper Plant By Waste Paper
- Mini Paper Plant From Eucalyptus Wood
- Mini Paper Plant From Jute Sticks & Wheat Husk Rice Husk
- Paper & Paper Products
- Paper (E.C.G. & E.E.G.)
- Paper And Paper Board From Jute Sticks
- Paper Bags For General Use
- Paper Bags For White Cement Bags
- Paper Board Manufacturing Unit
- Paper Cones & Tubes
- Paper Cones & Tubes (Automatic Plant)
- Paper Cups For Ice Cream
- Paper Envelops
- Paper From Bagasse
- Paper From Bamboo
- Paper From Rice Husk & Wheat Husk
- Paper From Waste Paper (Cap 40 Mt/Day)
- Paper From Waste Paper, Bamboo Chips Rice & Wheat Husk
- Paper From Wood Pulp Bamboo Etc.
- Paper Napkin, Facial Paper & Toilet Roll From Tissue Paper
- Paper Napkins & Air Mail Paper
- Paper Plate With Silver Lamination
- Paper Plates
- Paper Plates With Silver Lamination.
- Paper Shopping Bag
- Poly Coated Paper
- Printed Paper Shopping Bags
- Printed Shopping Bags.
- Pulp From Bamboo Wood
- Self-Sealing Paper Envelopes
- Silicon Release Paper
- Silicone Coated Paper
- Straw Board (Automatic Plant) From Rice Husk & Bagasse
- Sundried Board From Waste Paper & Pulp
- Tissue Paper
- Tissue Paper, Toilet Paper & Air Mail Paper Roll
- Tracing Paper
- Wall Paper
- Writing & Printing Paper
- Writing & Printing Paper Plant

Pesticides, Insecticides & Allied Products

- Aerosol insecticide Spray
- Ayurvedic Gamexane (Using Red Moing)
- Bagon Spray
- Boot Polish
- Copper Oxychloride
- D.D.T. Powder
- Grease Manufacturing Unit
- Mosquito Coil And Mats
- Mosquito Coils
- Mosquito Mats And Liquids
- Mosquito Repellant Candle
- Mosquito Repellant Liquidator
- Mosquito Repellant Oil
- Mosquito Repellant Mats
- Mosquito Repellant Agarbatti
- Pesticide Formulation
- Pesticides
- Phenyl (Black & White)
- Phenyl Pine Oil Disinfectants
- Urea Formaldehyde Resin

Petroleum, Waxes & Allied Products

- Anti-Static Lubricating Oil Used For Polyester Fibre Spinning
- Automatic Candle Making Plant
- Bees Wax
- Bio Gas Power Plant.
- Bitumen Emulsion Cationic Type.
- Bitumen.
- Bituminous Felts For Water Proofing And Damp Proofing
- Brake Fluids [Dot-3 Type)
- Brake Oil, Coolant & Packaging Of Lubricant Oil & Grease
- Break Oil
- Calcined Petroleum Coke
- Candle Making Plant (Semi Automatic)
- Candle Making Unit (Automatic)
- Chlorinated Paraffin Wax (CPW)
- Coaltar Distillation
- Coloured Flamed & Perfumed Candles
- Coloured Flamed Candles (Red, Blue & Green)
- Compound Wax From Residual Oil
- Coolant & Brake Oil
- Cough Syrup
- Crude Oil Refinery (Like Gasoline, Diesel, Jet Fuel, LPG, Kerosene & Bitumen)
- Cutting Oil
- Feldspar
- Furnace Oil
- Grease & Lube Oil From Used Engine Oil
- Grease Manufacturing
- Grease Manufacturing (Calcium, Lithium & Sodium)
- Grease Used For Chasis
- Jute Batching Oil
- Liquid Shoe Polish
- Lube Oil From CNSL Reduce

WE CAN PREPARE

PROJECT REPORT

ON ANY ITEM AND INDUSTRY OF ANY SCALE OF YOUR CHOICE

Market Survey Cum Detailed Techno Economic Feasibility Report on All Above Projects are Available. Contact :

NIIR PROJECT CONSULTANCY SERVICES

AN ISO 9001 : 2000 COMPANY

106-E, Kamla Nagar, Delhi - 110 007. Ph.: 23843955, 23845886, 23845654 Mob.: 9811043595 Fax : 91-11-23841561

E-mail : npcs.india@gmail.com / info@ niir.org Website : www.niir.org